Where Lt. Colonel Weinstein has been featured:

Fitness Magazine
The History Channel
Fox Sports Net
Fox News Channel - Fox & Friends
The Washington Times
The Las Vegas Tribune
Eurosport TV
Gold Coast Magazine
Tropical Life Magazine Miami
The Sun-sentinel South Florida
The Miami Herald
USA Today
Oxygen Magazine
Univision
Telemundo
RAZOR Magazine
Boca Raton Magazine
Comcast Newsmakers
Army Times
Go Riverwalk Fort Lauderdale
WSFL The Morning Show
NBC Nonstop Miami
NBC6 South Florida Today
New Times Broward-Palm Beach
Navy League News - Fort Lauderdale Council
The Navy Leaguer
SoBeFit Magazine

"The successful warrior is the average man with laser-like focus.

                                        - Bruce Lee

BOOT CAMP SIX-PACK ABS

Abdominal Training for All Fitness Levels

**Lt. Colonel Bob Weinstein
U.S. Army, Retired
Boot Camp Fitness Instructor**

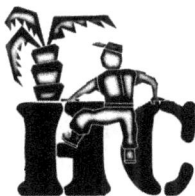

**Health Colonel Publishing
www.BeachBootCamp.net**

**Colonel Bob's Blog:
ColonelBobsBeachBootCamp.blogspot.com/**

Boot Camp Six-Pack Abs: Abdominal Training for All Fitness Levels
By Lt. Colonel Bob Weinstein, US Army, Retired.
Note: Bob is the nickname of Lt. Colonel Joseph R. Weinstein, US Army, Ret.
www.BeachBootCamp.net
Categories: physical fitness, health and fitness, abdominal exercises, calisthenics, boot camp fitness, boot camp workouts, army boot camp

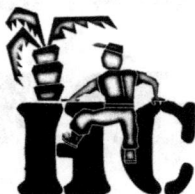

Health Colonel Publishing
The Health Colonel Series™

ISBN-13: 978-1-935759-17-1
ISBN-10: 1935759175
Library of Congress Control Number: 2012913358

Before beginning any exercise program, consult your physician. The author and publisher of this book and workout disclaim any liability, personal or professional, resulting from the misapplication of any of the training instructions described in this publication.

Weinstein, Bob.
Boot Camp Six-Pack Abs: Abdominal Training for All Fitness Levels
/ by Bob Weinstein, Lt. Colonel, US Army, Ret..– 1st ed.
ISBN-13: 978-1-935759-17-1 (trade pbk. : alk. Paper)
1. Fitness, Exercise, Abdominal Exercises–United States. I. Weinstein, Bob.
Weinstein, Joseph. II. Title. III. Boot Camp Six-Pack Abs

Printed in the United States

BOOT CAMP SIX-PACK ABS

Abdominal Training for All Fitness Levels

Lt. Colonel Bob Weinstein
U.S. Army, Retired
Boot Camp Fitness Instructor

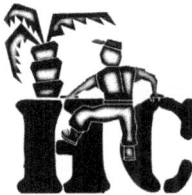

Health Colonel Publishing
www.BeachBootCamp.net

Colonel Bob's Blog:
ColonelBobsBeachBootCamp.blogspot.com/

"The successful person makes a habit of doing what the failing person doesn't like to do."

- Thomas Edison

ACKNOWLEDGEMENTS

Many thanks to all the
beach boot camp recruits on Fort Lauderdale Beach.
You remain a constant source of inspiration.
I thank you for your friendship and camaraderie.
May you prosper and enjoy a healthy and happy life.
I thank the Harbor Beach Marriott Resort & Spa on Fort
Lauderdale Beach in South Florida
for allowing me to use their property.
A special thank you goes to my wife, Grit,
who supports me in all that I do. She appears in many of
the Swiss ball exercises. Thank you to TJ Gillespie for
the great photos. Thank you Denise Zacharias for the
great photos. You will see TJ perform the very advanced
exercise called the Dragon Flag.

Photography by TJ Gillespie
www.DreamingInPhotography.com

Being fit and healthy has nothing to do with eating or exercise and has everything to do with how we think.

Boot Camp Six-Pack Abs

CONTENTS I

Boot Camp Six-Pack Abs

CONTENTS II

Boot Camp Six-Pack Abs

CONTENTS III

INTRODUCTION

This is your opportunity to exercise some of those important core muscles, the abdominals. You will find military exercises as well as other useful abdominal exercises. Though this book is focusing on abdominals, your approach to physical fitness should always be a complete body workout to include the cardio. Cardiovascular training is the most important form of exercise and you can find ways to combine working your strength and muscle endurance while working your cardio by getting your heart rate up for a duration of time.

Many diseases are related to the fact that the organs in your body are not getting enough oxygen. Cardiovascular training will help you to prevent such diseases, such heart disease, diabetes, stroke and many others. Why am I mentioning cardiovascular training in a book about abdominal workouts? What's the use of great abs if you cannot enjoy them due to diseases brought on by lack of cardo? I think you can answer that question.

Maintain a complete body approach and always be health focused when exercising. And, by the way, keep it fun.

Bob Weinstein
Lt. Colonel, U.S. Army, Retired
www.beachbootcamp.net

HOW TO USE THIS BOOK

You are interested in improving your abdominals and you may be interested in a clearly visible six-pack at some point in your training. The first goal of improving your abs is a worthy one. The second goal of achieving visible, six-pack abs is not a worthy goal and may not be healthy, long-term. Whether your abs become visible at some point in your training will depend on your body type and your calorie management. Even if you should have a body type that makes visible abs possible, it still may not be a healthy state for your body. Your abs do not need to be visible to be well trained.

Some of the exercises in this book are for all fitness levels, others are more advanced. Some of the more advanced exercises can be safely modified while you develop your muscles to be able to complete the full range of motion. Use the workout plans and seek out a workout buddy to help keep you on track.

Staying fit and healthy is a long-term goal, not one that comes and goes based on how you feel. A health-focused exercise program is not the same as a more advanced athletic program or one that focuses on appearance. Make sure that you are adjusting your lifestyle to include exercise, healthy eating and healthy thoughts so that you may more fully enjoy life and have more energy to help others and work more productively.

There are enemy soldiers on America soil. The names of these soldiers are Heart Disease, Cancer and Stroke. They are killing over 3,000 Americans a day.

PART A

BASIC ABDOMINAL EXERCISE INFO

Ground Rules to Succeed

1. Know the who, what, why, how, when and where.
Get your plan together and don't worry if it is incomplete. Action is preceded by planning. Some of the details of that goal are gathered while you are on the move to achieve your goals. This journal serves the purpose of helping you to keep the who, what, why, how, when and where covered as you pursue your journaling journey to better health. A poem by Rudyard Kipling says it best:

> *"I keep six honest serving-men*
> *(They taught me all I knew.)*
> *Their names are What and Why and When*
> *And How and Where and Who."*

2. Never give up if the cause is worthy.
Better health is a worthy cause. Therefore, never ever give up. Sir Winston Churchill said it best:
> *"Never give in--never, never, never, never, in nothing great or small, large or petty, never give in except to convictions of honour and good sense."*

3. Go around, through, over and / or under all obstacles.
There will be obstacles along the way. Deal with them and overcome them. There will be interruptions, set-backs, and thoughts of "I don't feel like it." that will invade the mind.

4. Inject Vitamin "D" for Discipline into your plan.
Include a good dose of D for discipline to keep you on track when you don't feel like it.
5. Take personal responsibility for your situation.
Never blame external circumstances or other people. That will keep you empowered to improve.

PART A - BASIC ABDOMINAL EXERCISE INFO

Goals - Three-Step Action Plan

1. Acknowledge and RECOGNIZE that there is a problem.
Has your "deviant" eating habits and lack of exercise become a lifestyle? Acknowledging and recognizing the problem appears to be easy to accomplish. It is easy because there is no action required other than acknowledgement and recognition. As Albert Einstein once said, *"Insanity is doing the same thing over and over again and expecting a different result."* If we are acknowledging and recognizing the problem with the forethought that no action is required, it is bogus and does not count. It is not genuine. Motives do matter and the motive with forethought that no action is required will not bring about the positive change you are looking for.

2. DECIDE when and how you are going to take action.
Decide when you will start and how you will take action.

3. Take ACTION.
Get up and start working on your goals now. Get up in the morning and start writing down all that you eat and drink. Write down your exercising routines. Move and allow momentum to overcome inertia.

PART A - BASIC ABDOMINAL EXERCISE INFO

WORLD RECORD AB EXERCISES

There are many categories of world records for abdominal exercises. I will name a few:

George Hood, who served as a marine, is famous for his Guinness World Record of one hour 20 minutes and 5.01 seconds holding the plank position. In December 2011.

The most sit-ups performed in 30 hours is 133,986, performed by Edmar Freitas in March of 2002.

Jack LaLanne, who passed away at the age of 96 in 2011, completed 1,033 sit-ups in 23 minutes.

Richard Hazard held the plank position for 50 minutes and 11 seconds.

Mark Pfelz managed to knock out 45,005 sit-ups in 58.5 hours in 1986.

PART A - BASIC ABDOMINAL EXERCISE INFO

MYTHS ABOUT AB EXERCISES

There are many myths about ab exercises. Here are just a few of them:

Myth #1: Equipment is needed to work the abs.

No equipment whatsoever is needed to work the abs. Militaries around the world have been training for centuries without special equipment. Why is that? Because it works.

Myth #2: Working the abs will reduce belly fat.

It is really hard to fight this myth due to all the advertising to the contrary. Please fight back and keep this answer in mind: No. Working the abs will <u>not</u> reduce belly fat no matter how much you perform abdominal exercises.

Myth #3: A six-pack is possible for anyone.

A <u>sustainable</u> six-pack is not possible for everyone without compromising health. We all have different body types. Cardio burns fat and fat reduction takes place everywhere regardless of the body part you are exercising.

Myth #4: Results are only possible with high reps.

Results are possible many different ways. Try reducing the reps and slowing the pace while pausing in the contracted abs position or perform push-ups or go for a run.

Myth #5: Ab muscles are unique.

Ab muscles are no different than other muscles in the body. There are both slow and fast twitch muscles in the body. Genetics will determine how many fast and slow twitch muscles you have.

PART A - BASIC ABDOMINAL EXERCISE INFO

US ARMY SIT-UP TEST

How do you measure up according to military standards? The sit-up chart below will let you know how you stand. The US Army requires that soldiers achieve a score of at least 60%. Some elite units have higher standards. To test yourself correctly, you must complete as many standard sit-ups as you can in two minutes. Correct form must be maintained and you are only allowed to rest in the up position. As soon as you stop the exercise with your shoulders on the ground, the test is terminated and your sit-up count is tallied Please note that the Army sit-up standard for men and women are the same. The chart below is depicting the age group 27 - 31.

LEVEL	MEN	WOMEN
ONE	21 - 32 REPS	21 - 32 REPS
SCORE	34 - 46%	34 - 46%
TWO	33 - 41 REPS	33 - 41 REPS
SCORE	47 - 62%	47 - 62%
THREE	48 - 60 REPS	48 - 60 REPS
SCORE	63 - 76%	63 - 76%
FOUR	61 - 72 REPS	61 - 72 REPS
SCORE	77 - 89%	77 - 89%
FIVE	73 - 82 REPS	73 - 82 REPS
SCORE	90 - 100%	90 - 100 %

Source: US Army Physical Fitness Test (APFT) Standards, effective 2012

PART A - BASIC ABDOMINAL EXERCISE INFO

ALTERNATIVE AB EXERCISES

There are many different abdominal exercises and most of them can be safely modified. Therefore, you will always have alternatives for working on the abs as long as they are approved by your physician if you should have medical issues or you feel pain or excessive discomfort.

Examples:

Crunches. Perform a partial crunch if you find you need to do so for medical reasons or simply because you are too fatigued to perform the full range of motion.

Sit-ups. If you are not able to perform a regular sit-up, you can attempt one and struggle to raise your upper body to the point you can achieve and then lower it back down. With time, your muscles will develop to the point that you will be able to complete the full range of motion as long as there are no medical reasons for not doing so.

MUSCLE CHART

MAJOR MUSCLE GROUPS

The Major Skeletal Muscles of the Human Body

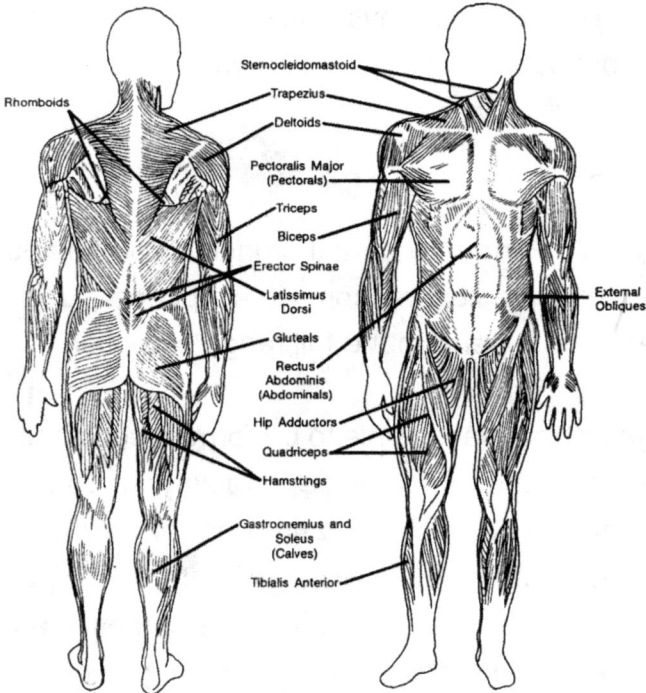

Sternocleidomastoid
Rhomboids
Trapezius
Deltoids
Pectoralis Major (Pectorals)
Triceps
Biceps
Erector Spinae
Latissimus Dorsi
External Obliques
Gluteals
Rectus Abdominis (Abdominals)
Hip Adductors
Quadriceps
Hamstrings
Gastrocnemius and Soleus (Calves)
Tibialis Anterior

The iliopsoas muscle (a hip flexor) cannot be seen as it lies beneath other muscles. It attaches to the lumbar, the pelvis, the vertebrae and the femur.

PART A - BASIC ABDOMINAL EXERCISE INFO

ABDOMINAL EXERCISES AS PHYSICAL THERAPY

Consider abdominal exercises as a form of physical therapy. Exercise is considered the best way to treat back problems and disk injury according to Consumer Medical Reports. The abdominal muscles consist of four muscle groups. These muscle groups are the internal oblique, external oblique, rectus abdominus and transversus abdominus muscles. They support organ stability, help in flexion and rotation of the trunk and they stabilize the trunk. Strong abdominal muscles support the skeletal frame and reduce the chances of back injuries.

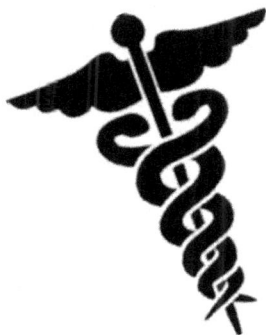

LOWER BACK PAIN

Performing abdominal exercises without maintaining a balance of exercises in your core area can result in lower back problems or may exacerbate injuries you may already have.

Consult with your physician if you are experiencing lower back pain. Remember to modify any exercise that seems to be overburdening due to injury or weakness of some muscles or perhaps due to imbalance.

DOES FORM MATTER?

As a general rule, exercise form does matter. Focus on proper form is designed to maximize the use of those muscles which are to be worked for a particular exercise and to maintain good body mechanics. Sometimes, maintaining proper form has the further purpose of preventing injury.

There is, however, a greater principle than form that needs to be applied. That principle is movement. Movement is more important than form as long as you are not injuring yourself. Most body weight exercises can be safely modified. In some cases, modifying an exercise is done to prevent injury. For example, if someone has problems with their knees, it may be advisable to modify the squat so that injury does not occur. Modifying the squat by only performing a partial motion would then allow for continuous work of the muscles without injury.

Many who attend my beach boot camp classes cannot perform regular sit-ups. I recommend partial sit-ups which means raising the body partially instead of going all the way up or simply struggling to raise the upper body during each repetition. This allows you to continue strengthening the muscles needed to perform a full range of motion sit-up.

PART A - BASIC ABDOMINAL EXERCISE INFO

CORE STRENGTH IS KEY

A mindset needs to change when it comes to working the core and, in particular, the abdominals. The predominant, false mindset is to think specifically about performing exercises that focus on the abdominal muscles. This mindset is false because all the muscles of the human body move in orchestration. Therefore, any exercises or drills that take advantage of the complete or predominant orchestration of the muscles, promotes muscle balance and good body mechanics which will help prevent injury when moving the body in activities of daily life, sports and physical activity at work.

Some examples of activities and exercises that recruit and work the core and therefore the abdominal muscles:

Running and sprinting.

Interval training.

Agility training.

Squats.

Push-ups.

Pull-ups.

Swimming.

Volleyball.

Football.

Tennis.

Zumba.

Water skiing.

PART A - BASIC ABDOMINAL EXERCISE INFO

MUSCLES WORKED

This is an example of the muscles worked when performing abdominal exercises. The fitness industry may use the categories of primary and secondary muscles. However, the muscles work in orchestration which means that simply because certain muscles are designated as being worked as a secondary muscle does not mean that - from a health standpoint - you are not getting a sufficient workout of those muscles as well. We may like to think in terms of isolating certain muscles when working out, our bodies respond in terms of muscles operating just the way the human body was designed to work, in concert.

Exercise	Primary Muscles	Secondary Muscles
Crunches	Rectus Abdominus	Abdominal Oblique
Sit-up	Rectus Abdominus	Tensor Faciae Latae
		Rectus Femoris
		Sartorius
		Abdominal Oblique
V Sit-up	Rectus Abdominus	Tensor Faciae Latae
		Pectineus
		Sartorius
		Rectus Femoris
		Abductor Longus
Twisting Crunch	Abdominal Oblique	Rectus Abdominus
		Psoas Major

MUSCLE IMBALANCE

Understand that exercise is about maintaining balance. Imbalance can result in injury and issues with your lower back. Muscles work in orchestration with. A boot camp program is designed to allow for your muscles to work together to create and maintain that balance. A complete body workout will generally keep your muscles in balance and in synch. Your core area, to include your abs and lower back are also being worked in running drills, jogging, squats and many other exercises. Not only are you getting an abdominal workout by performing those exercises you will find in this book, but when you are performing many other exercises that are a part of a complete body workout.

PART A - BASIC ABDOMINAL EXERCISE INFO

ABDOMINAL EXERCISES FOR WOMEN

The are several great abdominal and core exercises for women.

Upper abs.

You can work the upper abs with crunches on an exercise ball or by performing elbow planks.

Obliques.

Bicycle crunches are great for the obliques.

Lower Abs.

Reverse curls will work wonders on your lower abs.

Most, if not all abdominal exercises for men are great for women too.

PART A - BASIC ABDOMINAL EXERCISE INFO

Are you looking for medical insurance? Make your premium payments in the form of living a healthy lifestyle void of dependence on a home pharmacy of medications.

PART B

ABDOMINAL EXERCISES

CRUNCHES

Lie down on your back and bend both knees with your feet on the ground. Clasp your hands behind your head or place them in a crossed position on your chest. Raise your shoulders slightly from the ground and lower them back down. That is one repetition. Perform 1 - 5 sets of 30 to 50 repetitions each.

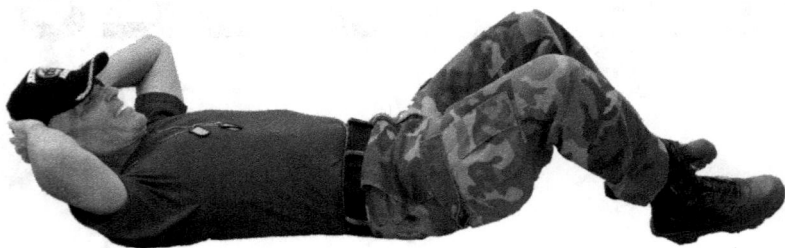

CRUNCHES

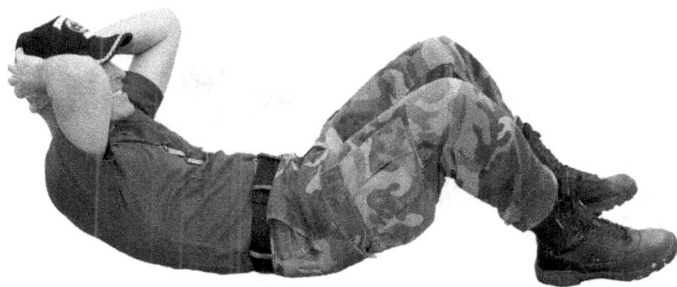

SAND BAG CRUNCH

Lie on your back with knees bent. Firmly hold weighted plate or other item, such as a sandbag behind your head or across your chest. Contract your abs and raise your upper body while keeping your lower back on the bench and raising your upper body as high as possible. Then return to the starting position with your shoulder back on the bench. Perform 3 - 5 sets of 10 to 40 repetitions each. Add more weight or less, depending on your level of strength and endurance.

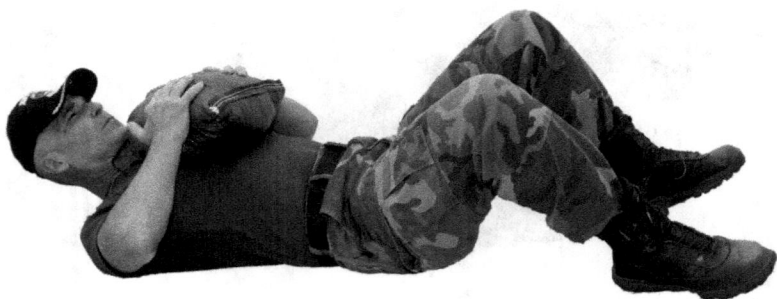

SAND BAG CRUNCH

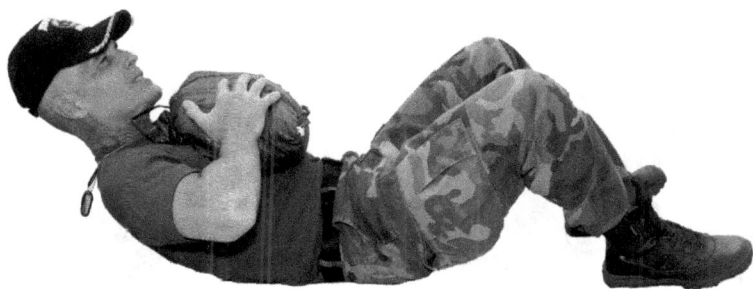

PART B - ABDOMINAL EXERCISES

CRUNCHES WITH LEG RAISED AND EXTENDED

Vary the crunch by doing crunches with one leg extended off the ground. Start out with the right leg extended six inches off the ground and hands still clasped behind your head. Practice a set of 30 reps on each leg. Perform 10 crunches with the leg six inches off the ground, then 10 with the leg half way up, then 10 with the leg in a vertical position. Now switch and do the same with the left leg or simply switch legs between each set of 10 reps with each leg.

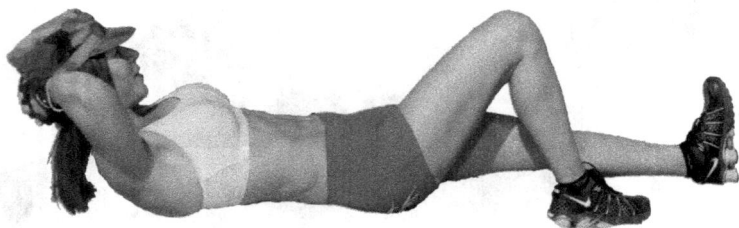

PART B - ABDOMINAL EXERCISES

CRUNCHES WITH LEG RAISED AND EXTENDED

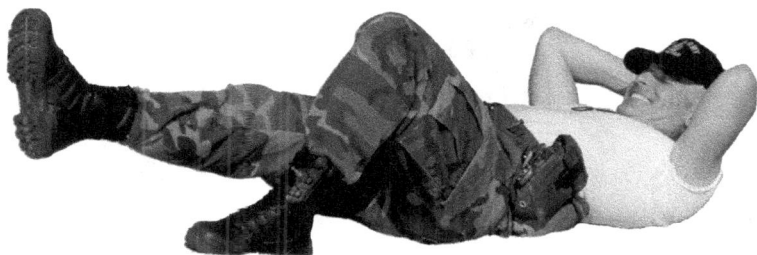

ALTERNATING ELBOW CRUNCH

Here's another great abdominal exercise. We'll call it the alternating elbow crunch. You're on your back. Your hands are clasped behind your head. Your left leg is bent. Cross your right leg over your left knee. Take your left elbow and reach for your right knee and back down. That is one rep. Use a smooth motion. Don't be concerned if you can't reach your leg with your elbow. Do the best you can. Remember, by performing the exercise you are working those muscles! Now switch off by crossing your left leg over your right knee, reach for your knee with your right elbow and do it again.

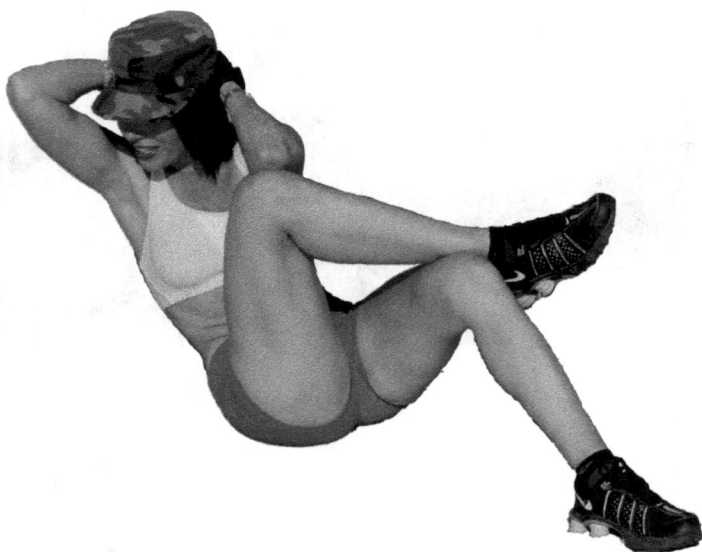

ALTERNATING ELBOW CRUNCH

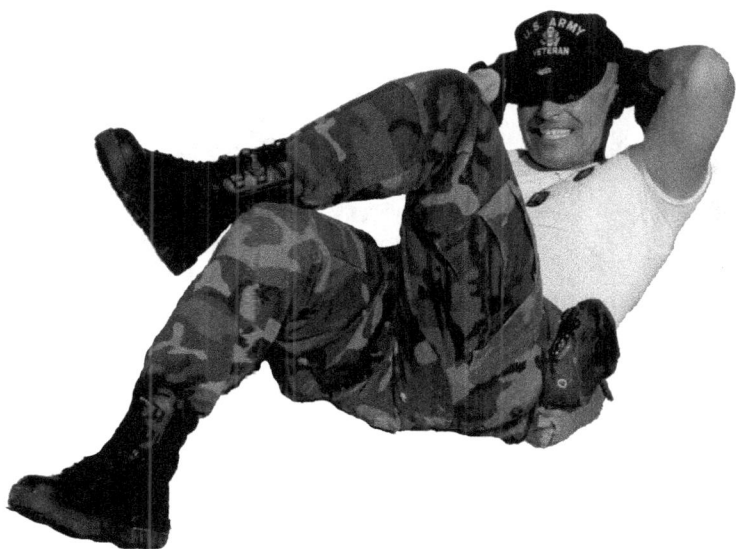

PART B - ABDOMINAL EXERCISES

CRUNCHES WITH ARMS VERTICAL

Lie on your back with arms extended in a vertical position and elbows locked. Raise your shoulders slightly off the ground and then back down. Remember to keep your elbow locked and maintain the vertical position with your arms. Do not rock forward with your arms. Maintaining the vertical arms position will focus the exercise on the abdominal muscles. Perform a crunch in this position. Perform 2 - 5 sets of 20 to 50 repetitions.

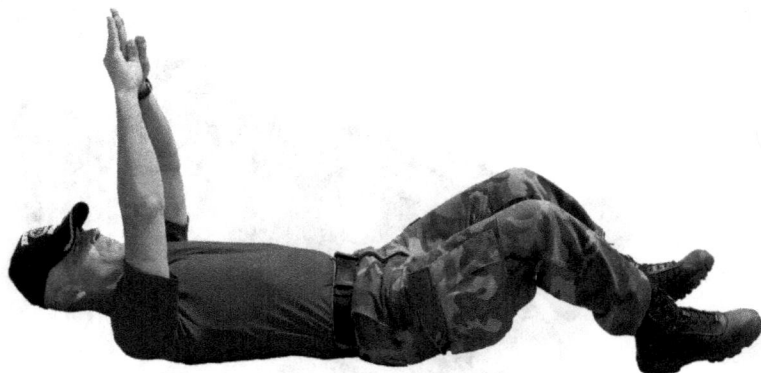

PART B - ABDOMINAL EXERCISES

CRUNCHES WITH ARMS VERTICAL

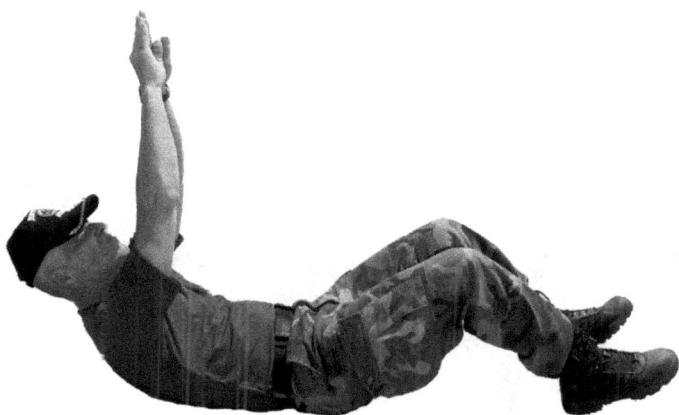

PART B - ABDOMINAL EXERCISES

REVERSE CRUNCH

Lie on your back with your knees bent and hands clasped behind your head. While maintaining your knees bent in the 90 degree angle, lift your legs to where your lower legs (from knees to feet) are parallel to the ground. You may increase the reverse crunch by raising your butt while crunching your lower body in the direction of your upper body. Perform 2 - 5 sets of 10 to 30 repetitions.

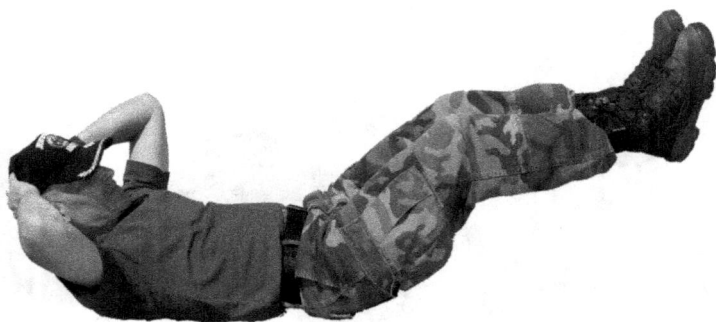

REVERSE CRUNCH

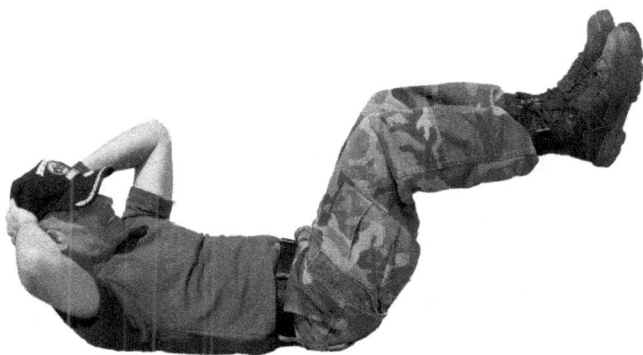

PART B - ABDOMINAL EXERCISES

HEEL PUSH CRUNCH

Get in the regular crunch position on your back with the knees bent and the hands behind your head. Raise your shoulders and press your heels into the floor. Do not pull on your neck. Simply support your head slightly. Perform Lower 10 - 40 repetitions of 2 to 5 sets.

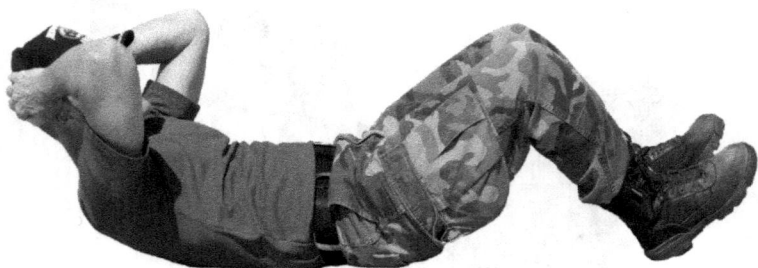

PART B - ABDOMINAL EXERCISES

HEEL PUSH CRUNCH

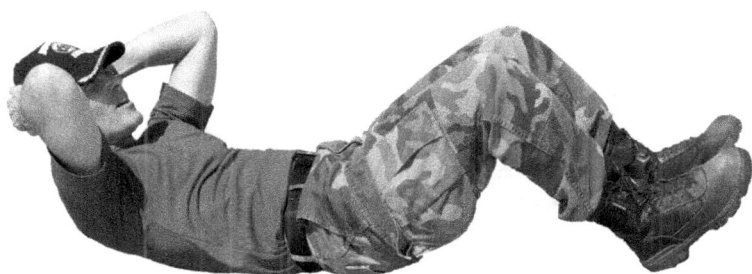

PART B - ABDOMINAL EXERCISES

VERTICAL LEGS CRUNCH

Lie on your back with legs extended in a vertical position and your feet crossed. Place your hands behind your head without pulling on your neck. Contract your abs and raise the shoulders a few inches and lower them back down. That is one repetition. Perform 10 - 40 repetitions of 3 to 5 sets.

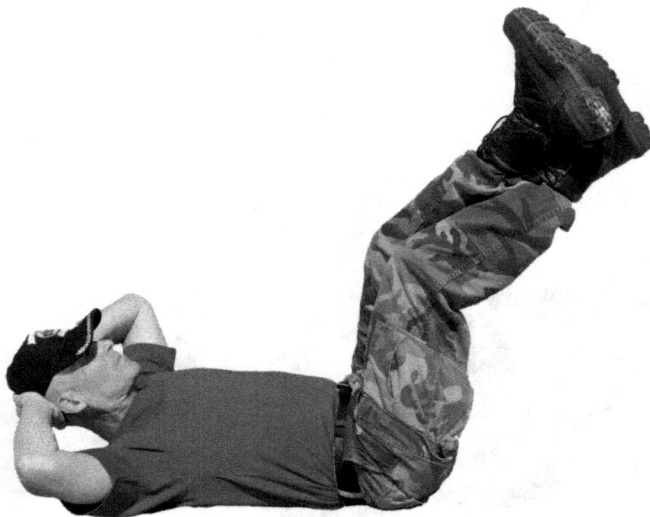

PART B - ABDOMINAL EXERCISES

VERTICAL LEGS CRUNCH

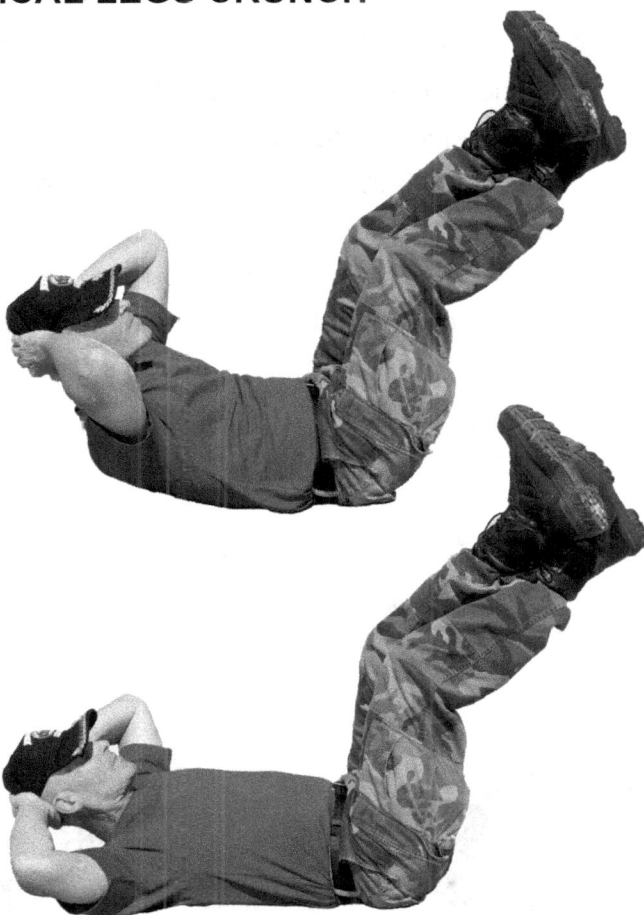

LONG ARM CRUNCH

Lie on your back and extend the arms straight out behind your head in an approximate horizontal position. While contracting your abs raise your shoulders at least 6 to 8 inches. Maintain your arms in a straight position. Try not to use your neck muscles which will avoid straining your neck. Perform 3 - 5 sets of 10 to 40 repetitions. You can increase the workout by making this a weighted exercise with a dumbbell.

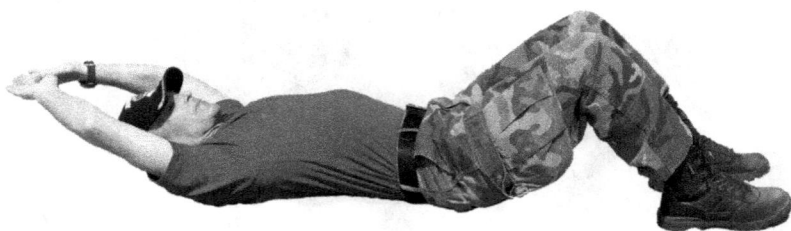

PART B - ABDOMINAL EXERCISES

LONG ARM CRUNCH

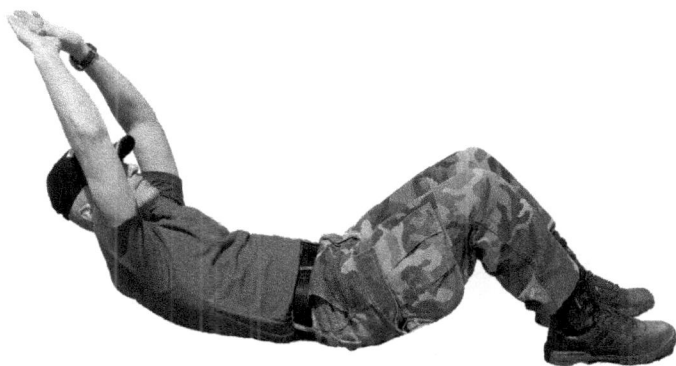

KNEELING CRUNCH WITH RESISTANCE BAND

Place the middle of your resistance band over a doorknob or use the accessory door attachment that came with your resistance band. Kneel down in front of the doorknob, grasp the each handle of your resistance band with a hand with palms facing downward and forearms facing upward. Bend your elbows at the level of your shoulders. Contract your abs and crunch your upper body downward with neck straight while lowering arms to chest. Perform 3 - 5 sets of 10 to 20 repetitions each.

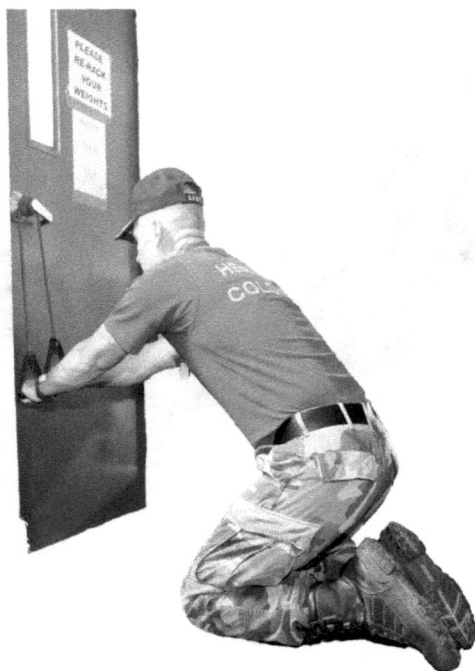

PART B - ABDOMINAL EXERCISES

KNEELING CRUNCH WITH RESISTANCE BAND

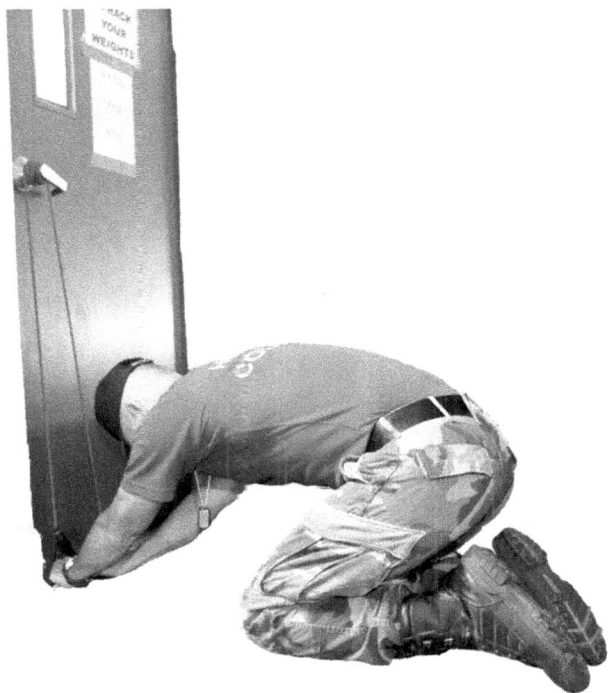

PART B - ABDOMINAL EXERCISES

KNEELING CRUNCH WITH CABLE

Set your appropriate weight, face the machine, grab the cable and kneel down facing the machine. Contract your abs and lower your body by pulling the cable down while keeping your arms extended and using your upper body to pull downward. Do not use the arms to pull downward. Push the cable down while arms are in a static position as depicted in the photo. Depending on the weight you use, perform 3 to 5 sets of 10 to 30 repetitions each.

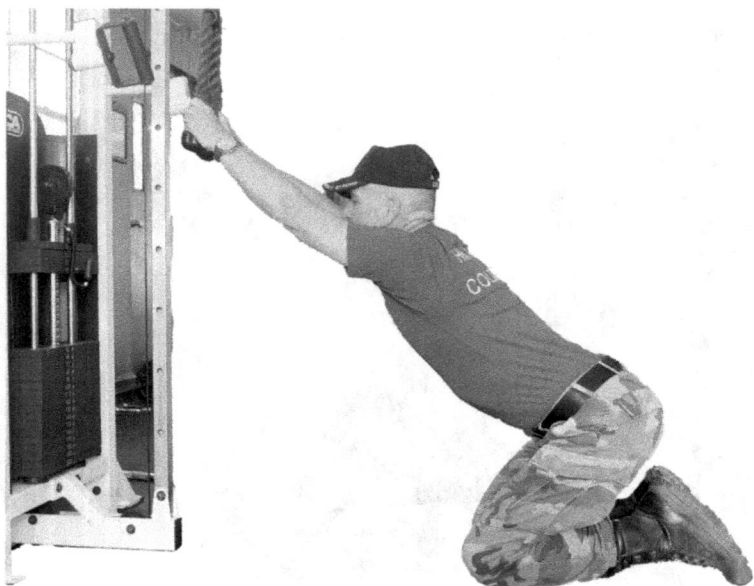

PART B - ABDOMINAL EXERCISES

KNEELING CRUNCH WITH CABLE

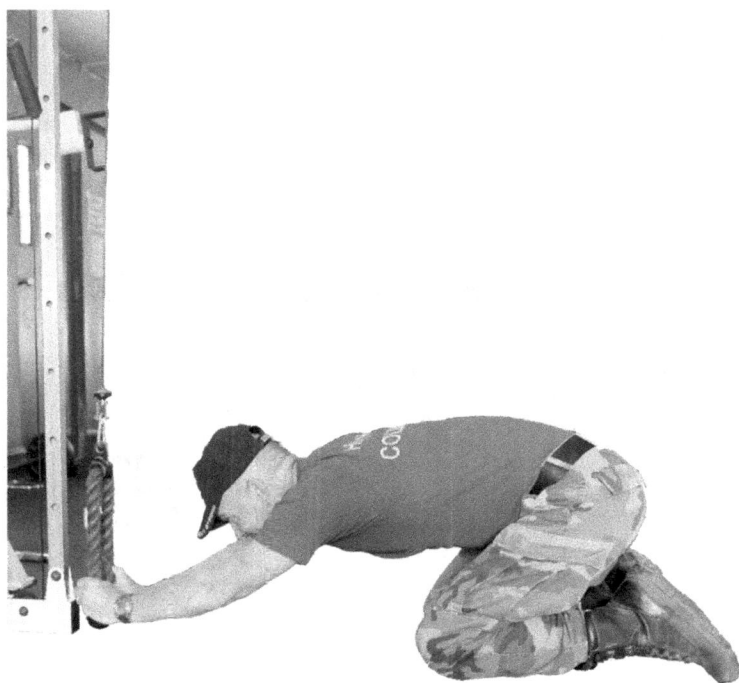

PART B - ABDOMINAL EXERCISES

SWISS BALL CRUNCH

Using a Swiss Ball, lie on the ball by placing it under your lower back. You may position your arms crossed behind your head or crossed over your chest. Lift your upper body off the ball while contracting your abdominals. Keep the ball steady while you curl up. The ball must remain stationary. Lower your upper body back down. Perform 1-5 sets of 15 to 30 repetitions each.

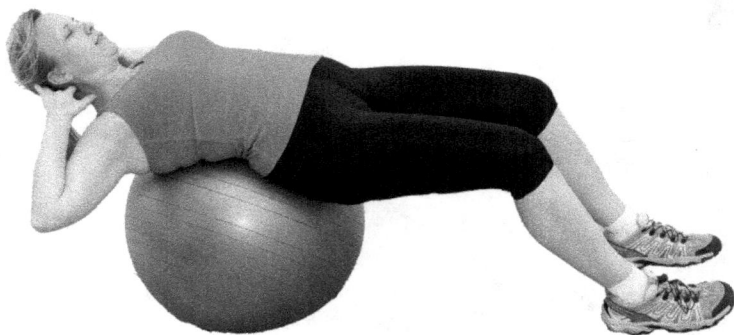

PART B - ABDOMINAL EXERCISES

SWISS BALL CRUNCH

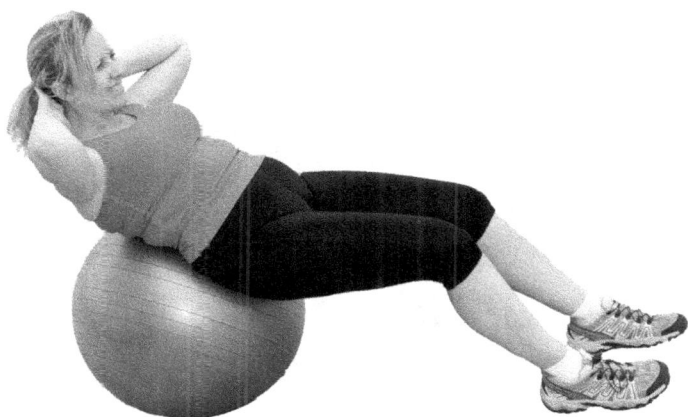

TWISTING CRUNCH WITH SWISS BALL

Sit on the ball and then gradually walk your legs forward and lie back on the ball until your shoulders and head are hanging off the ball with your knees and hips bent. Bend your body so that your back is contoured over the ball. Contract your abs to raise your upper body while twisting your upper body in one to the right and return to the starting position. You may alternate by twisting your upper body to the right and then the left or your can perform all your repetitions of a set by twisting to one side only and then the same number of reps for the other side.

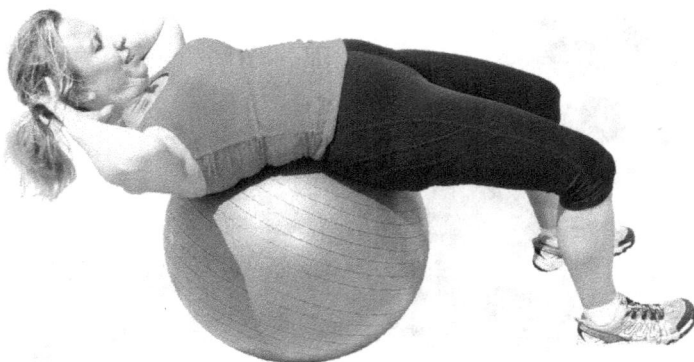

TWISTING CRUNCH WITH SWISS BALL

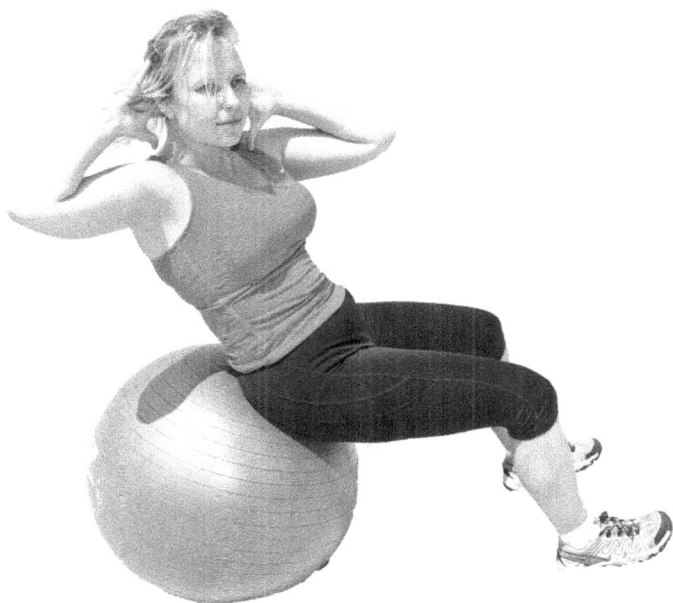

MEDICINE BALL TWISTING CRUNCH

Lie on your back with both knees bent and your feet on the ground. Hold your medicine ball at chest level with both hands and contract your abdominal muscles. Lift your shoulders to a partial sit-up position and swing the ball to your right side at the same time while counting to three and then return to the starting position on a count of four and repeat for the other side. One repetition is a four count on one side. Use even numbers of repetitions. Perform 6 - 20 repetitions of 3 to 5 sets.

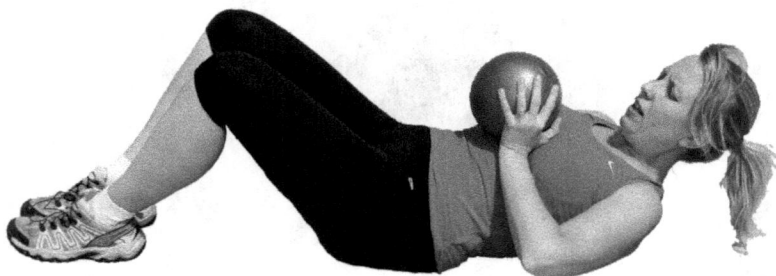

PART B - ABDOMINAL EXERCISES

MEDICINE BALL TWISTING CRUNCH

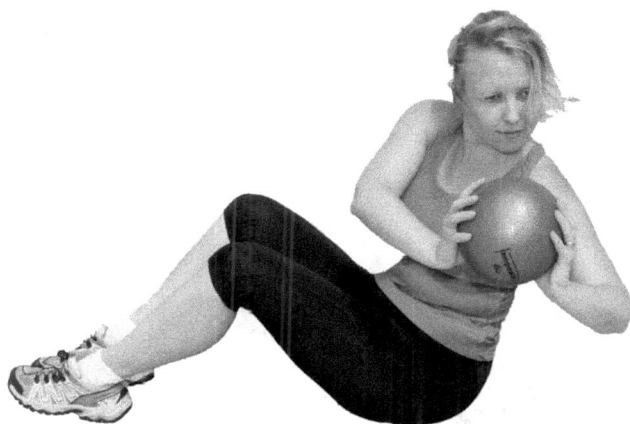

PART B - ABDOMINAL EXERCISES

LYING SWISS BALL CRUNCH

Lie down on your back with your knees bent and your feet flat on the ground. Place the exercise ball between your knees and grasp it with your knees. Raise the ball with your legs while pressing your back down and contract your abdominals. You may place your hands across your chest in a crossed position or place them behind your head. Lift your shoulders off the ground and raise your hips slightly off the ground and hold for two seconds, then roll back down to the starting position with a controlled motion. Do not use momentum as this will diminish the workout. Remember, this is a small motion. Perform 3 - 5 sets of 10 to 30 repetitions each.

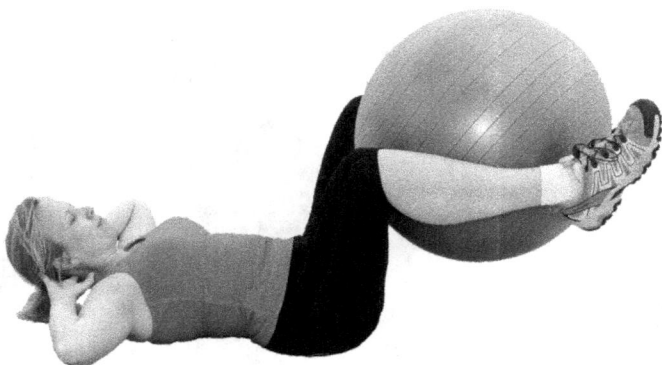

LYING SWISS BALL CRUNCH

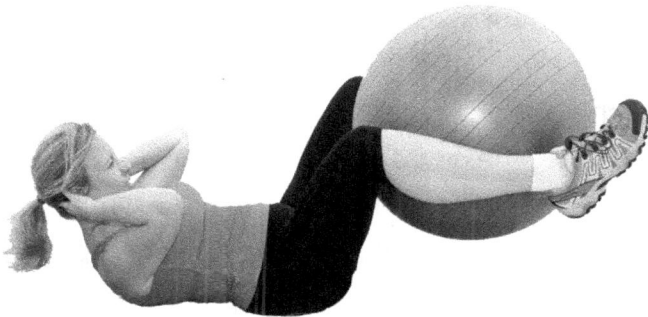

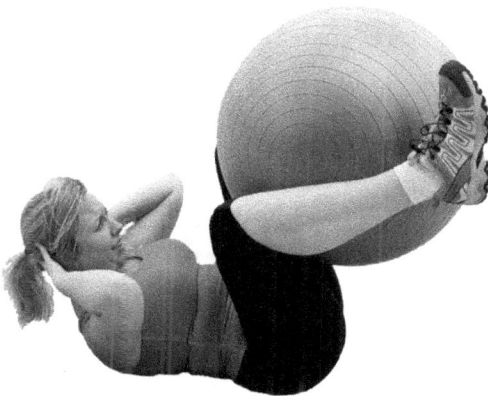

ARMS STRAIGHT UP SWISS BALL CRUNCH

Position your body on the exercise ball with your ball placed under your lower back, bend your hips slightly and position your legs at a 90 degree angle with feet on the ground and placed less than shoulder width apart. Move your back over the curve of the ball and extend your arms straight up. Contract your abdominals and gluts. While keeping your neck straight, crunch your upper body forward and then back to the starting position. Make sure your hips do not move off the ball. Use a controlled motion for this exercise. Perform 1 - 3 sets of 5 to 20 repetitions each. If you find you are losing your balance, stop, recover and then start again.

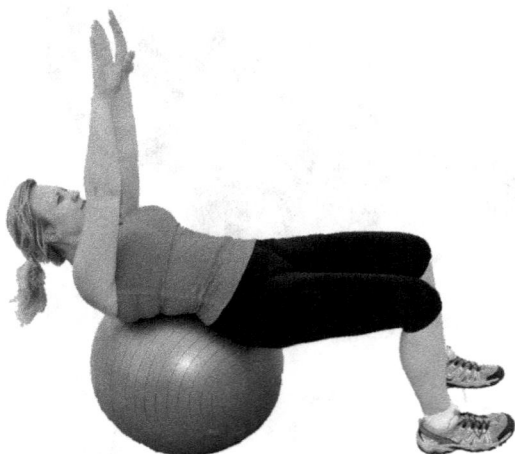

PART B - ABDOMINAL EXERCISES

ARMS STRAIGHT UP SWISS BALL CRUNCH

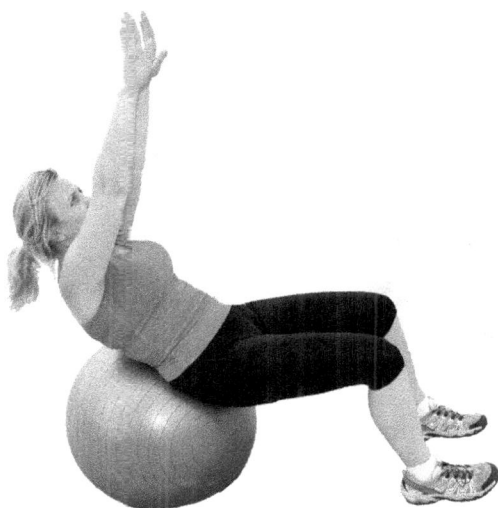

SIT-UP

The sit-up is great for strengthening the abs and hip-flexors. Lie down on your back with your arms across your chest or hands clasped behind your head and knees bent. You may use a buddy to hold your ankles or place your feet under a sturdy object to keep your feet on the ground during the exercise or you can perform it without leg support. With a smooth motion, raise your upper body to the vertical position or beyond and then lower it back down while allowing your spine to roll smoothly back down to the starting position. Perform 3 - 5 sets of 40 to 100 repetitions each.

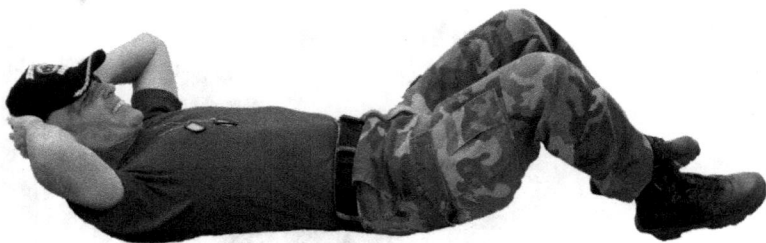

SIT-UP

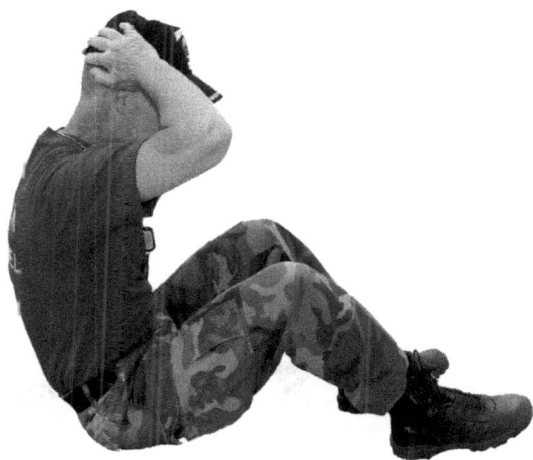

PART B - ABDOMINAL EXERCISES

V SIT-UP

The V sit-up is performed as follows: Lie on your back with your arms extended over your head in a horizontal position. Raise your legs and upper body so that they form a V in mid-air and lower them back down. That is one repetition. This is a more advanced exercise and do not be concerned if you find you are struggling. Struggle with a partial motion if necessary. Keep practicing and those muscles will eventually develop and you will gain better balance in the upper position. Perform 3 - 5 sets of 10 to 30 repetitions each.

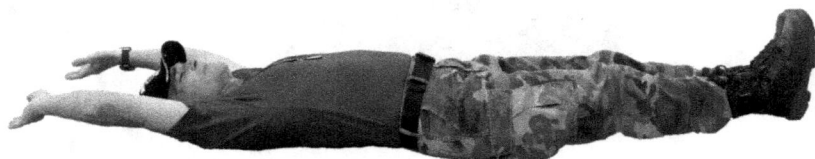

V-SIT UP

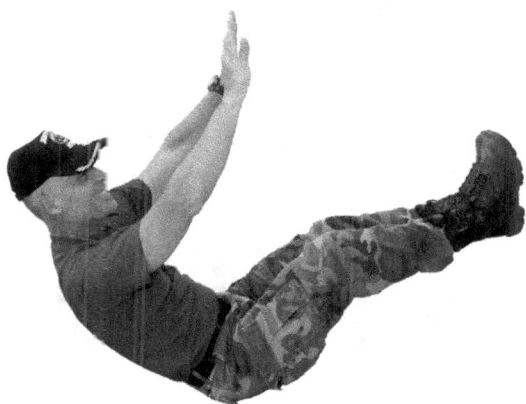

PART B - ABDOMINAL EXERCISES

ATOMIC SIT-UP

With the atomic sit-up we are now going nuclear. Just kidding. Some think this is an exercise from the Cold War. Lie down on your back with legs extended and arms extended to your sides. The starting position is with legs six inches off the ground and extended. Now pull your knees and your chest to the middle where you are in a position balanced on your butt. Your body is briefly in that jack-knifed position. As you move into this position, bend your elbows so that your hands are at your shoulders. Now lower your legs back out to the extended position with feet six inches off the ground with your arms extended. That is one repetition. You may need practice before your body can perform this exercise. Perform 3 - 5 sets of 10 to 20 repetitions each.

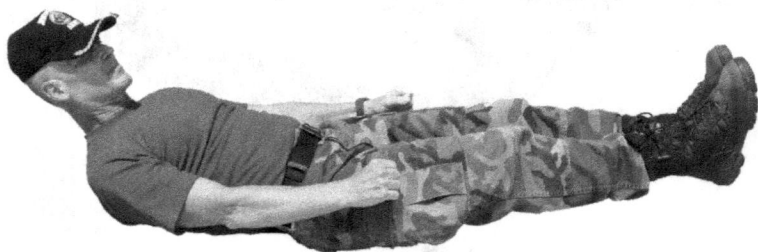

ATOMIC SIT-UP

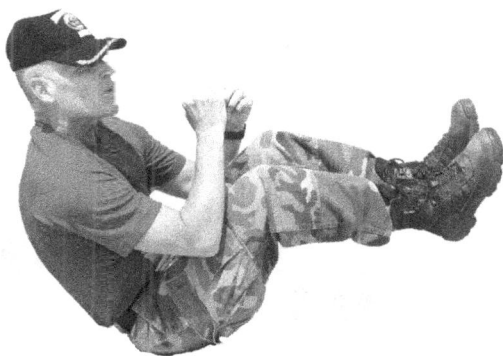

TWISTING SIT-UP

The twisting sit-up is an advanced form of sit-up. You can either use an incline sit-up bench or perform them on the floor. Lie on your back with hips and knees bent. Place hands behind your neck or across your chest. Raise your upper body and twist to one side. Return to the starting position and repeat, alternating the twist to the other side. Perform 3 - 5 sets of 10 to 20 repetitions each.

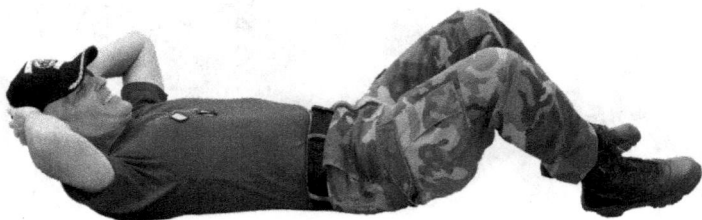

TWISTING SIT-UP

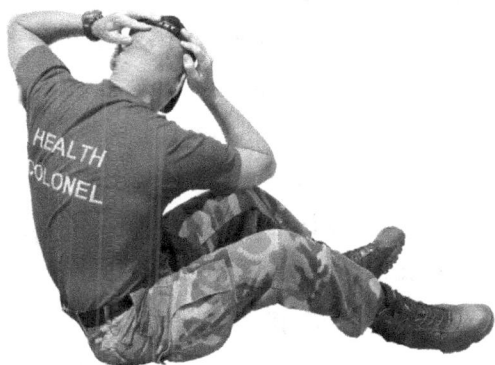

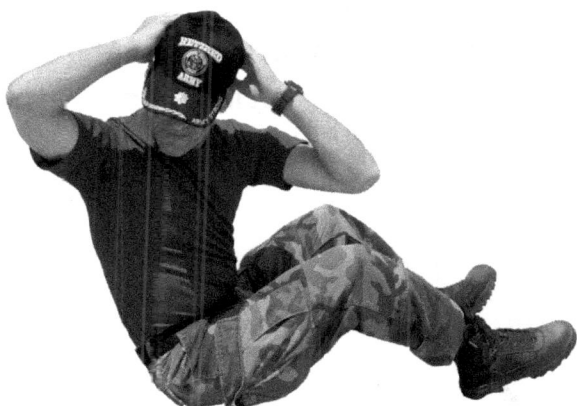

FOUR COUNT LEG LEVERS

Place your hands with palms facing down on the ground and arms extended at the sides of your body to stabilize the lower back with your head raised. The starting position is with legs raised six inches off the ground and together. Now here is the four-count. ONE – raise the legs up to about 36 inches off the ground. TWO – spread the legs while still raised at the 36 inch level. THREE – bring the legs back together while still at the 36 inch level. FOUR – back down to the position six inches off the ground with legs together. This exercise also works the hip flexors, lower abs and lower back. Perform ten reps per set with multiple sets. Start off with no more than five reps per set if you notice a lot of strain on the lower back and work up to ten reps.

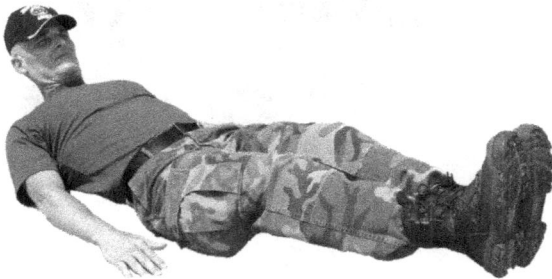

PART B - ABDOMINAL EXERCISES

FOUR COUNT LEG LEVERS

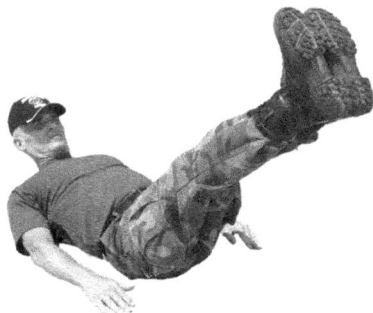

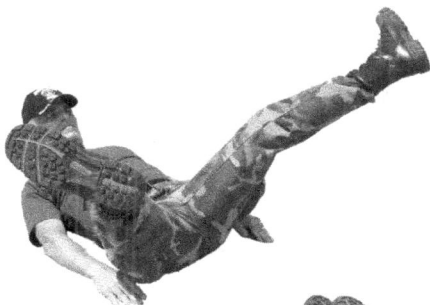

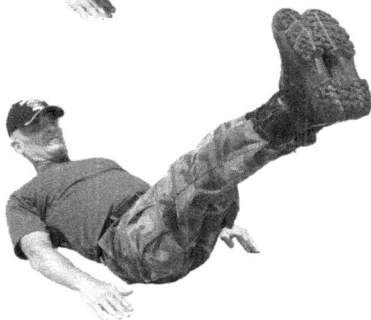

FLUTTER KICKS

Lie on your back with arms extended on the sides of your body and palms facing down on the ground to stabilize the lower back with your head raised. Raise both of your legs in a staggered position (one leg is higher than the other) with a slight bend in the knees. This is a four count exercise. With each count you will simply switch the leg positions which makes it look like a scissor move, not bicycle pedaling. This is your leg movement for the count: ONE, scissor move; TWO, scissor move; THREE, scissor move; FOUR, scissor move. Here's how you count the reps: One, two, three, ONE; one, two, three, TWO; one, two, three, THREE, one, two, three, FOUR; one, two, three, FIVE. Do five to ten reps per set with multiple sets and very brief rests between sets.

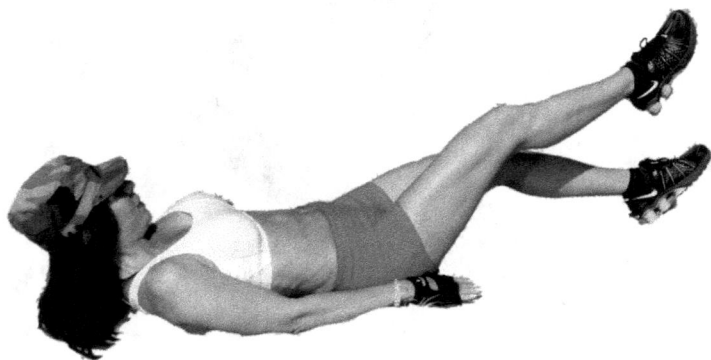

PART B - ABDOMINAL EXERCISES

FLUTTER KICKS

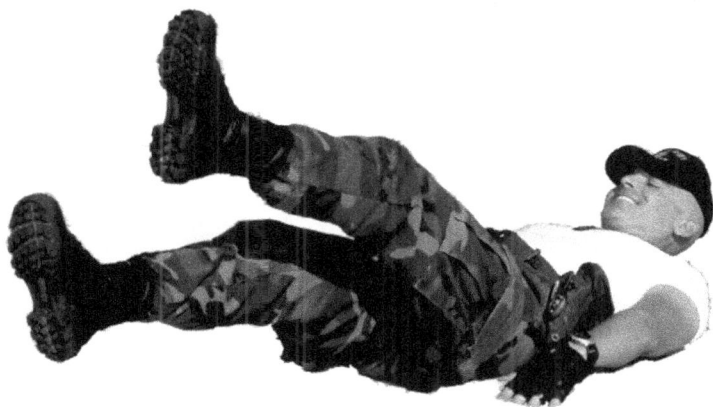

PART B - ABDOMINAL EXERCISES

DRAGON FLAG

This exercise became popular in the movie Rocky IV when Sylvester Stallone used this as a part of his training. The name Dragon comes from one of Bruce Lee's nicknames, "little dragon". Lie horizontal on a bench. Hold the underside of the bench with your arms to secure your shoulders to prevent your body from rolling forward. Pull the rest of your body up in the in the air in a diagonal position from the bench with only your hands and shoulder on the bench. Begin with the legs contracted and extend the legs slowly to increase the challenge of the movement since you are moving your weight farther from the point where you are holding the bench. Your knees and hips remain locked in the extended position while performing this exercise using the abdominals.

PART B - ABDOMINAL EXERCISES

DRAGON FLAG

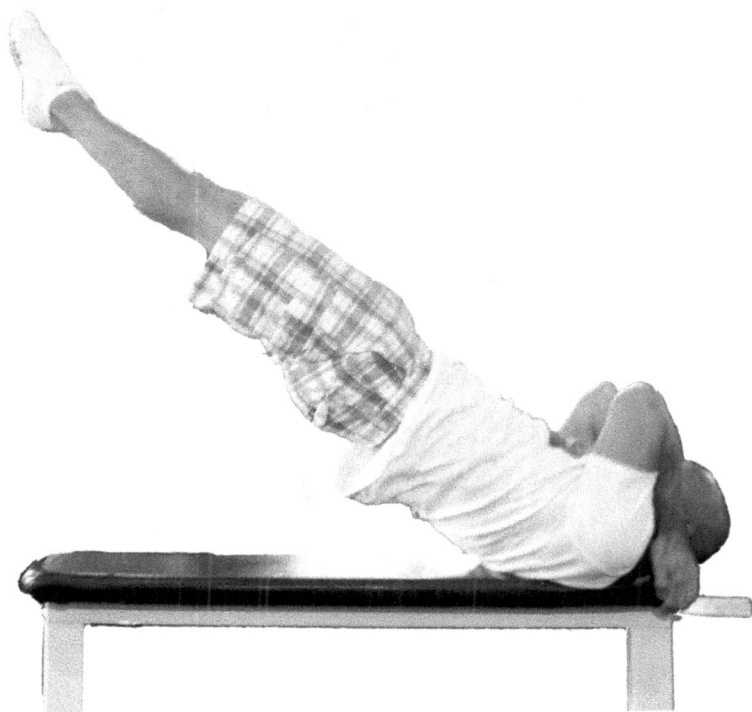

SIDE BENDS FOR OBLIQUES

Stand with your back straight, shoulders relaxed and feet about shoulder width on the floor. Place your right arm on your hip to the side. Place your left hand behind your head. Bend your waist to the right side. Then slide your right hand to the starting position. That is one repetition. Perform 2 - 5 sets of 10 to 40 repetitions. Reverse sides and perform the side bends again. You can alternate by performing, for example, 20 reps on the right side and then 20 on the left.

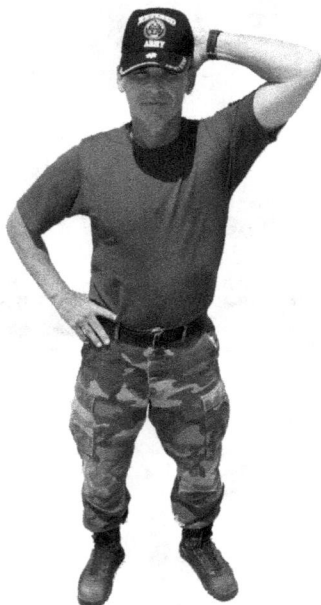

PART B - ABDOMINAL EXERCISES

SIDE BENDS FOR OBLIQUES

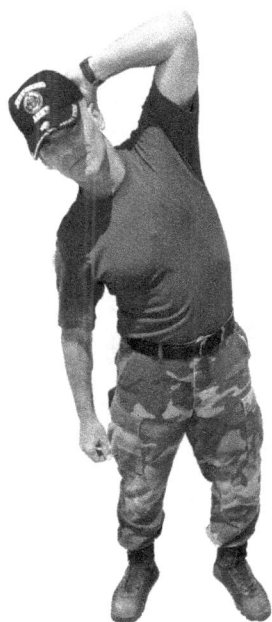

PART B - ABDOMINAL EXERCISES

SAND BAG SIDE BENDS

Stand with your back straight and feet should width apart. Hold your sandbag or dumbbell in your right hand with right arm extended to your side and palm facing your body. Place your left hand on your hip. While contracting your abdominal muscles, bend from your waist to the right as far as you can and return to the starting position. That is one repetition. Alternate sides with each set. Perform 20 - 5 sets of 20 to 50 repetitions.

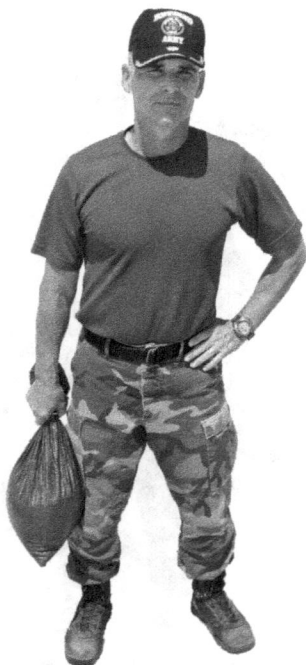

PART B - ABDOMINAL EXERCISES

SAND BAG SIDE BENDS

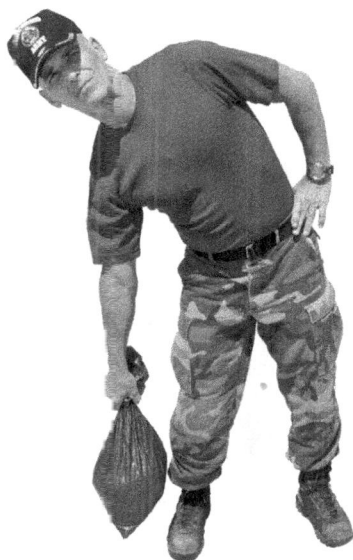

PART B - ABDOMINAL EXERCISES

MEDICINE BALL SIDE BENDS

Hold the medicine ball between your hands in front of your stomach in the standing position. Your feet are shoulder width apart. Contract your abs and raise the ball over your head with arms completely extended. While maintaining your arms in an extended position holding the ball and both feet on the ground, gradually sway your body over to the right side as far as you can without hurting yourself. Hold that position and count slowly to three and return to the starting position on the fourth count. Repeat the movement to the left side. Alternating between sides perform 10 - 20 repetitions of 3 to 5 sets.

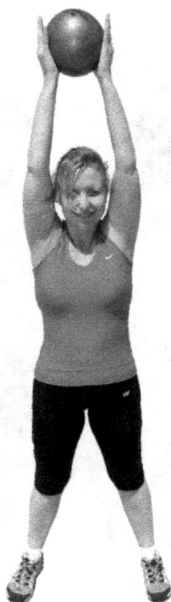

PART B - ABDOMINAL EXERCISES

MEDICINE BALL SIDE BENDS

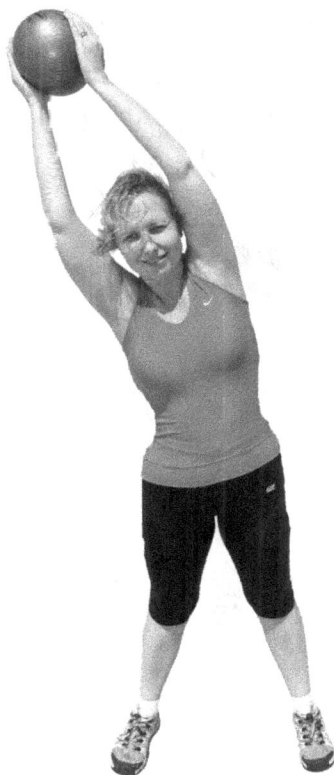

PART B - ABDOMINAL EXERCISES

SWISS BALL SIDE BENDS

You will need a Swiss ball for this exercise. Hold the ball between your hands in front of your stomach in the standing position. Your feet are shoulder width apart. Contract your abs and raise the Swiss ball over your head with arms completely extended. While maintaining your arms in an extended position holding the ball and maintaining both feet on the ground, gradually sway your body to the right side as far as you can without hurting yourself. Hold that position and count slowly to three and return to the starting position on a count of four. Repeat the movement to the left side. Alternating between sides perform 10 - 20 repetitions of 3 to 5 sets.

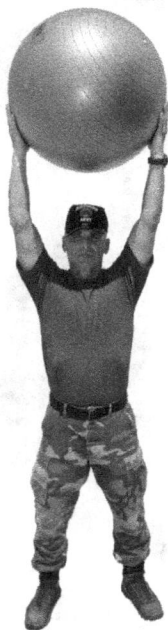

PART B - ABDOMINAL EXERCISES

SWISS BALL SIDE BENDS

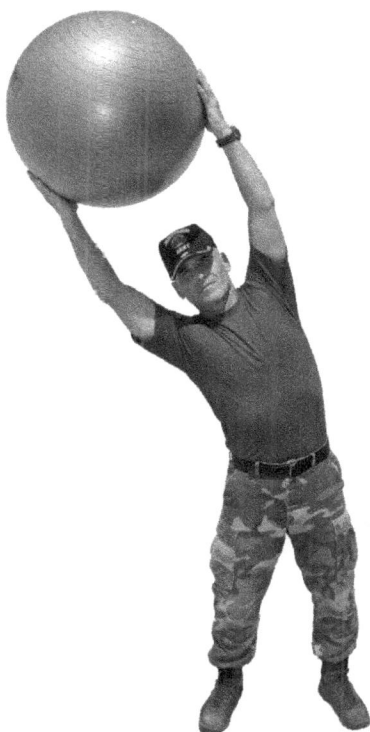

V ROCK AND ROLL

Lie on your back with your legs together and your feet and arms extended in a horizontal position with your hands together as if you were about to dive into water. Contract your abdominals and raise your legs, arms and shoulders at least 6 - 8 inches off the floor. Rock your body like a rocking chair back and forth. Each back and fourth rocking motion is one repetition. Perform 3 to 10 repetitions of 3 to 5 sets.

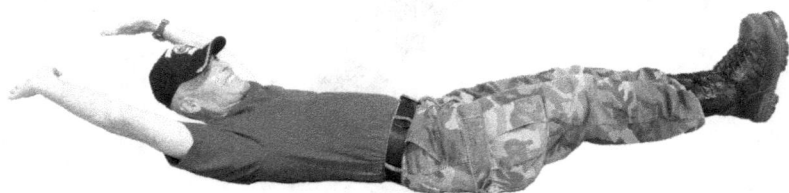

V ROCK AND ROLL

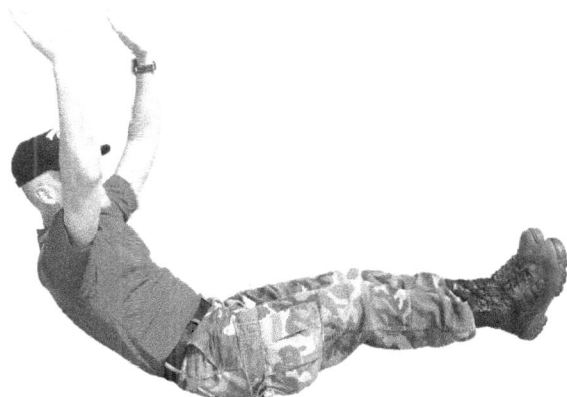

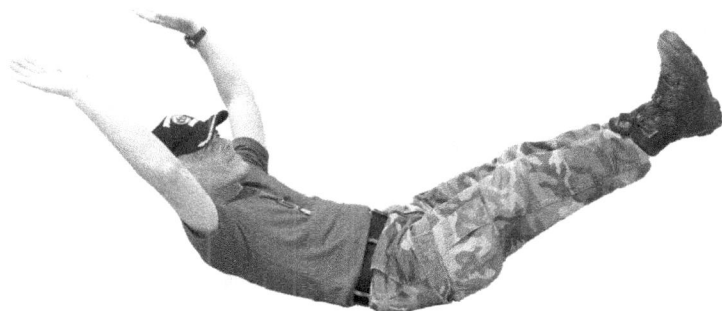

BICYCLE EXERCISE

Lie on your back with your hands behind your head. Raise your knees to your chest and lift your shoulders off the ground. That is the starting position. Rotate your shoulder area to your right as you raise your right elbow towards your left knee while you straighten your right leg and then switch to the other side. That is one repetition. Create the bicycle motion by switching sides. Perform 10 - 20 repetitions of 3 to 5 sets.

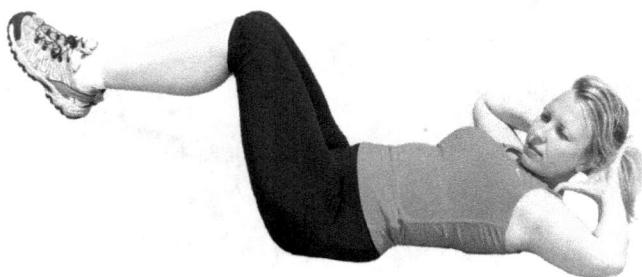

PART B - ABDOMINAL EXERCISES

BICYCLE EXERCISE

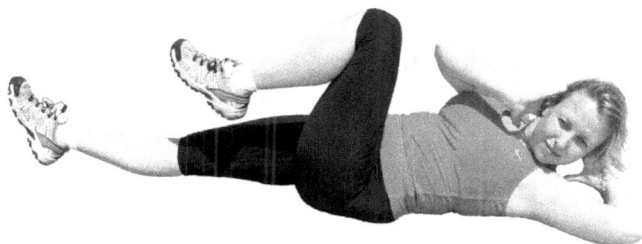

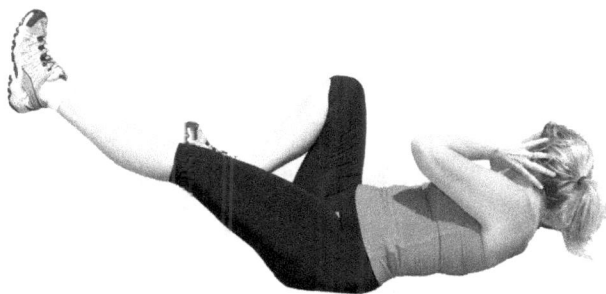

PLANK ON ELBOWS AND TOES

Get in the push-up position on the ground. Bend your arms so that you are supported by your forearms which are flat on the ground. You are now on your toes with your back straight and you are on your elbows. Contract your abdominals and hold the position for 20 to 60 seconds. Perform 3 to 5 repetitions.

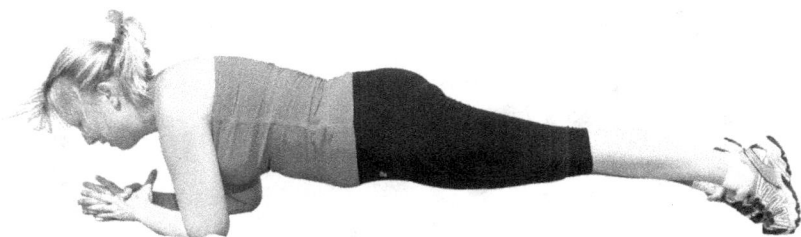

PLANK ON ELBOWS AND TOES

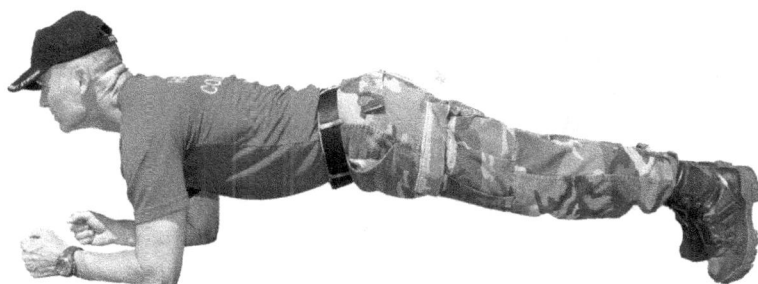

SIDE PLANK

Lie on your side on the floor. Place your forearm on the floor under your shoulder and perpendicular to your body. Your legs are extended with your upper leg on top of your lower leg. Raise your body so that it is completely straight and ridged. Hold that position for 20 to 30 seconds or raise and lower your body to perform repetitions. Switch sides and repeat. Perform 10 - 20

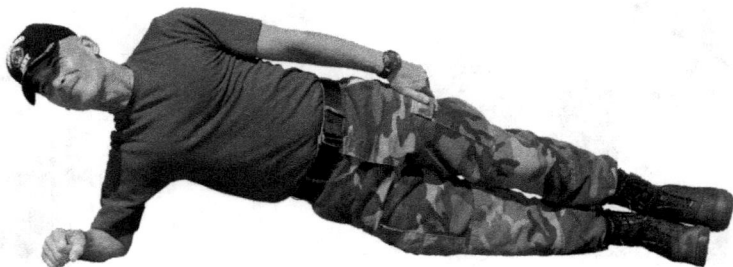

PART B - ABDOMINAL EXERCISES

SIDE PLANK

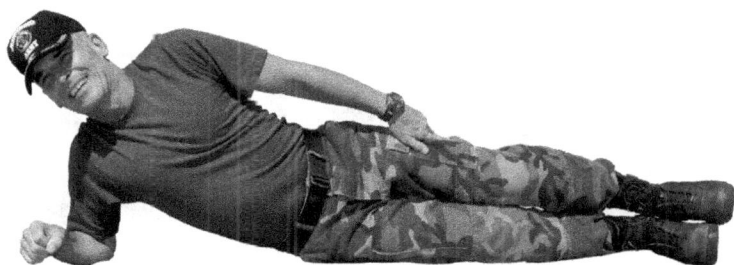

BUTT UPS

Get in the regular push-up position and instead of your arms in the regular position, place your elbows on the floor while resting on your forearms with your arms at a 90 degree angle.

Your back should be arched slightly and not straight as with a regular pushup. Arch your back slightly out rather than keeping your back completely straight.

Raise your butt upward while contracting your abs. It will look like you are forming a V with your butt in the air and upper and lower body straight. Then you will lower your body back to the starting position.

Perform 5 - 10 repetitions of 3 to 5 sets.

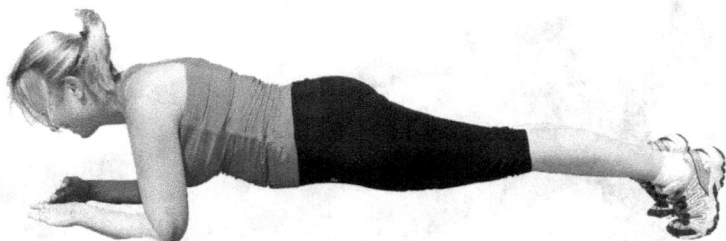

PART B - ABDOMINAL EXERCISES

BUTT UPS

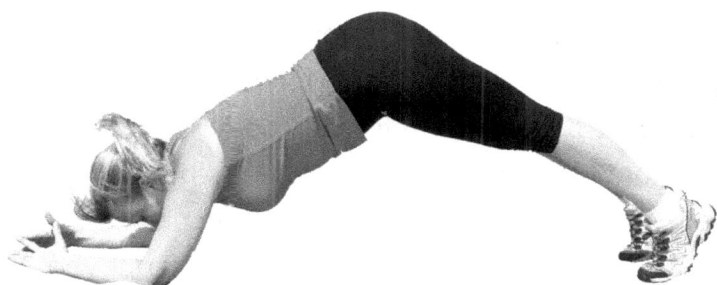

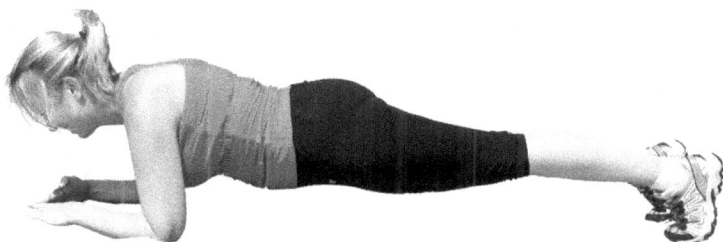

AB ROLLER

Kneel down on the floor and hold the ab roller by the handles in front of you on the floor. Your arms are straight in a vertical position and elbows locked and ab roller on the floor. While maintaining your arms straight and back rigid, gradually roll the ab roller forward as far as you can go without collapsing until your body is straight. Your body should not touch the floor. Hold the "out" position briefly and then roll back to the starting position.

Contract your abs during this exercise. If you have lower back problems, this exercise may not be advisable for you. You can add some variety by rolling out to the sides instead of straight forward.

Perform 10 - 25 repetitions of 3 to 5 sets. You can count the repetitions by counting "out" in the rolled out position and then "one" for the return position counting the first repetition.

AB ROLLER

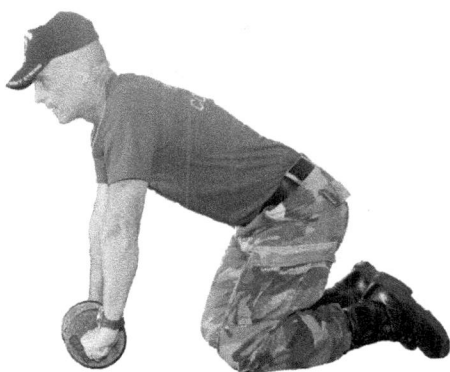

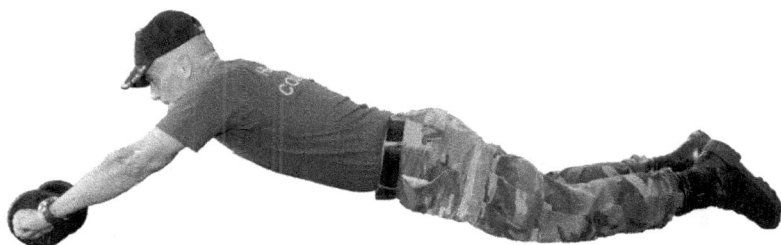

PART B - ABDOMINAL EXERCISES

SWISS BALL AB ROLLS

Kneel down in front of the Swiss ball and place your forearms and fists on the ball. Hold your abs contracted and your back straight but with a natural spine curvature. Roll forward gradually until you feel your abs completely engaged and then back to the starting position.

Stay in touch with your body. If you notice your back is overly burdened only go forward as far as you can without hurting yourself. You will swivel at your hips as you maintain your upper body rigid. Your arms and abdominals will be doing most of the work for this exercise.

Perform 5 - 15 repetitions of 1 to 3 sets.

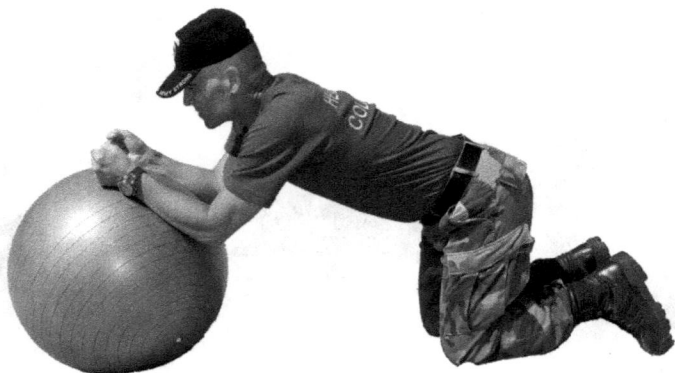

PART B - ABDOMINAL EXERCISES

SWISS BALL AB ROLLS

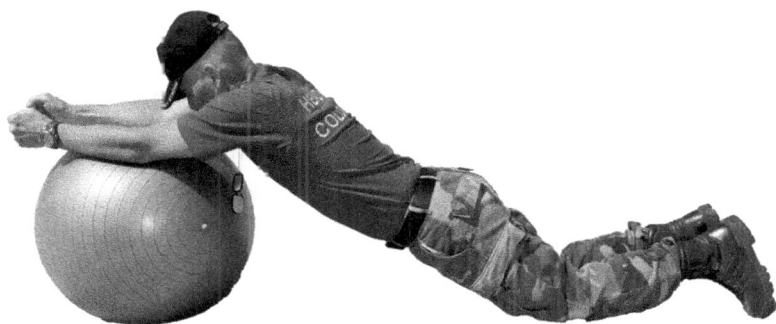

We have a health pollution crisis in this country.
We are polluting our health by how we live.

PART C

WORKOUT PLANS

10 WEEK
1,000 AB REPS / RUN PLAN

The purpose of this workout is to achieve maximum muscle endurance and strength with a combined jog / run and intermittent sets of abdominal exercises. to benchmark where you stand with your basic abdominal strength and endurance, test yourself by doing as many sit-ups or crunches as you can in two minutes. Test yourself once a week or every two weeks on an off day of training or before going for a run.

Your goal: Complete a total of 1,000 (or more) repetitions during a 60 minute jog / run without stopping.

How it's done: Drop down and knock out 30 to 50 regular ab exercise reps, get right back up and jog / run for 80 to 150 yards. Then get back down and perform the next set of abdominal exercises. You will continue this for 60 minutes and keep count of repetitions completed. Only stop briefly to drink water. Unless you already have excellent cardio and muscle endurance, you will not complete 1,000 repetitions within 60 minutes of a jog / run workout.

Your strategy:. As soon as you notice you cannot keep going with your exercise repetitions and run, modify the pace and reduce your repetitions per set before stopping. Instead of 50 repetitions per set, take it down to 20 or 30 per set as necessary.

Frequency: 3 to 4 times per week.

Exercise at least five days per week with mostly cardio.

PART C - WORKOUT PLANS

EXAMPLE:
TRAINING LOG
10 WEEK 1,000 AB EXERCISE REPS / RUN WORKOUT

Week	Reps	Sets	RPE
1	200	12	8
2	250	10	8
3	360	15	7
4	480	20	10
5	580	22	9
6	680	24	5
7	750	18	7
8	820	26	8
9	940	27	6
10	1000	30	7

NOTE: If you complete the 1,000 ab exercise reps before 60 minutes have passed, keep the abdominal exercises / run workout going until you have reached 60 minutes and record your score.

RPE stands for Rate of Perceived Exertion (see chart). You should stay within 60% to 80% of your Target Heart Rate. That would be an RPE of about 5 to 8, hard to very hard.

PART C - WORKOUT PLANS

1,000 SIT-UPS PURE

There are a few people who may be interested in doing 1,000 sit-ups without stopping in one super set. A workout program like this may be ambitious but is not necessarily healthy nor is it realistic to maintain.

Your body will need enormous muscle endurance and you will need to maintain your body strength balance by working all the muscles of the core, amount others. For those of you who are ambitious enough to try this one, remember, this is just for a challenge and not necessarily to promote health. To exercise for health does not require you in to engage in such a workout. Your connective tissue may be strained. Most of you will not achieve this goal no matter how much you train. And if you're training that much, what are you doing with the rest of your life?

Nine ways of thinking that could lead to your demise

Adopt a pill popping mentality.
Adopt a Can't-do-anything-to-change-it mentality.
Adopt a closed mind.
Failed to ask, "Am I doing all that's reasonably possible?"
Adopt a disregard cause-and-effect mentality.
Adopt a philosophy of sedentary lifestyle.
Adopt a disregard-what-is-most-important mentality.
Eat predominantly refined foods.
Think that BMI stands for Big Mac Injection.

PART C - WORKOUT PLANS

RPE OR RATE OF PERCEIVED EXERTION

RPE is an easy way to determine what level of exertion you are applying to your aerobic workout. In the fitness world we normally think of cardio (aerobic) and strength training as separate. Combining them will result in a new level of strength and cardiovascular conditioning. Your muscle strength training will add an important component called muscle endurance training, the ability of the muscle to continuously work while fatigued. Excellent muscle endurance is probably more important from a health standpoint than simply strong muscles. RPE is how you perceive the level of fatigue.

RPE SCALE	
0	Nothing at All
1	Very Weak
2	Weak
3	Moderate
4	Somewhat Hard
5	Hard
6	
7	Very Hard
8	
9	
10	Very, Very Hard

PART C - WORKOUT PLANS

PYRAMID WORKOUTS

Another great way to increase strength and endurance are with pyramid workouts. A pyramid workout with push-ups could, for example, be built by gradually increasing the reps for five sets and then gradually decreasing for four sets back to the starting number of reps. Pyramid workouts can be used for just about any exercise. Many times our bodies will plateau and not continue to make strength or cardio progress. The body has adapted to whatever routine we are doing. Pyramid workouts will interrupt your routine and cause your muscles to respond to strength and endurance improvements.

Example

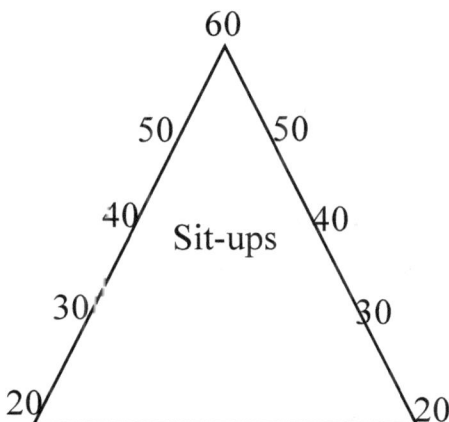

TIMED CIRCUIT TRAINING

Push-ups circuit training combined with abdominal exercises can be found in U.S. Army physical training manuals in many variations. As a timed event, this is excellent for groups or individuals. The trainer would keep time and call the exercises until you have completed all eight sets. If you are getting too fatigued to complete the particular exercise with the proper form, use a partial motion for the exercise so that you are still working those muscles until the trainer calls out to switch to the next one.

Timed sets are designed to increase strength and muscle endurance. You will probably feel some muscle soreness for a couple of days.

SET NO.	EXERCISE	DURATION	REST
1	Reg. Push-ups	30 Seconds	30 Seconds
2	Crunches	30 Seconds	30 Seconds
3	Tricep Push-ups	30 Seconds	30 Seconds
4	Sit-ups	30 Seconds	30 Seconds
5	Knee Push-ups	30 Seconds	30 Seconds
6	Flutter Kicks	30 Seconds	30 Seconds
7	Reg. Push-ups	30 Seconds	30 Seconds
8	Crunches	60 Seconds	End

MORE TIMED CIRCUIT TRAINING

This timed circuit training is a simplified version alternating between push-ups and sit-ups. You can also substitute the sit-ups with a different abdominal exercise such as crunches. If the times are too easy for you, make adjustments that work for you.

SET NO.	EXERCISE	DURATION	REST
1	Reg. Push-ups	40 Seconds	0 Seconds
2	Sit-ups	40 Seconds	0 Seconds
3	Reg. Push-ups	30 Seconds	0 Seconds
4	Sit-ups	30 Seconds	0 Seconds
5	Reg. Push-ups	30 Seconds	0 Seconds
6	Sit-ups	30 Seconds	0 Seconds

100 SIT-UPS
FIVE WEEK WORKOUT PLAN

For those of you who are interested in becoming one of the few who can perform 100 sit-ups in two minutes, this workout plan is for you.

Test: Benchmark where you are now at with sit-ups and perform as many as you can in two minutes. Whatever that score is, divide it in half. That will be your reps per set. If you tested with a score of 30 sit-ups, your training set will be 15 reps. Test yourself once a week and adjust your training reps accordingly.

Training Sets: Perform 10 sets per training day. Rest 20 to 60 seconds per set.

Training Days: 3 days per week, with rest days, if possible. A rest day means go do some cardio.

Optional: Supplement with crunches, 2 days per week, 10 sets per training day.

Optional: Mix pyramid training and the combined jog/run and sit-ups workouts.

If you have not accomplished your goal of 100 sit-ups after five weeks, repeat the last two weeks and keep working.

5 WEEK WORKOUT PLAN FOR 100 SIT-UPS
TRAINING LOG (ONE DAY)
EXAMPLE

Set Number	Target Reps	Actual Reps
Set no. 1	15	15
Set no. 2	15	15
Set no. 3	15	15
Set no. 4	15	12
Set no. 5	15	10
Set no. 6	25	9
Set no. 7	25	9
Set no. 8	25	8
Set no. 9	25	7
Set no. 10	25	5

This is an example of one day's entries. Notice the decrease in actual reps from one set to the next. The reason for this will probably be lack of sufficient muscle endurance to maintain the target reps. Do not be concerned about this if it happens to you. You are making progress because you are reaching the point of fatigue. From week to week your muscle endurance (and strength) will improve.

About the Author

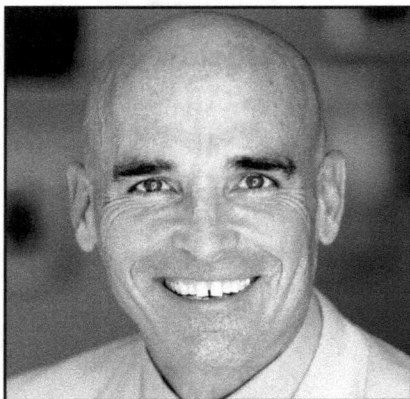

Joseph "Bob" Weinstein
Lt. Colonel, U.S. Army, Retired
www.BeachBootCamp.net
Blog: www.colonelbobsbeachbootcamp.blogspot.com/

BIO

Born in Washington, D.C., **Lt. Colonel. Bob Weinstein** grew up in Virginia and spent 20 years in Berlin, Germany; he is retired from the United States Army as a Lieutenant Colonel with 30 years of service and spent about half that time as a senior military instructor with the Command & General Staff College at one of the satellite locations in Germany.

He has been featured on radio and television, among others, on the History Channel and Fox Sports Net as well as in various publications such as the Washington Times, The Miami Herald and the Las Vegas Tribune.

His background is unique and diverse, including: military instructor, attorney, motivational speaker, wellness coach, certified corporate trainer, and certified personal trainer. He is fluent in German and English.

He is a popular motivational speaker at corporate events and banquets and conducts military-style workouts on Fort Lauderdale Beach utilizing strength, cardio, flexibility and agility training - both in personal training and group sessions.

He strongly believes in the importance of giving back to the community. Col. Weinstein has volunteered his time for homeless and run-away kids at the Covenant House and has devoted time to training youth who are members of the US Naval Sea Cadets Corps, Team Spruance, Fort Lauderdale, Florida.

He is a member of the American Council on Exercise.

He is the author of *Boot Camp Fitness for All Shapes and Sizes, Weight Loss - Twenty Pounds in Ten Weeks* and others. Some of his previous clients as a guest speaker include: Sony, DHL, American Express, KPMG, AOL, IBM, AARP, SmithBarney, Green Bay Packers and Humana.

Lt. Colonel Bob Weinstein
U.S. Army, Retired
954-636-5351
www.BeachBootCamp.net

"There are no hopeless situations, there are only people who have grown hopeless about them."

- Clare Boothe Luce

"He Ain't Heavy, He's My Brother."

The line "He ain't heavy, he's my brother," has been used for many decades now. That picture of one child carrying his or her brother is what comes to mind. Many artists have done versions of a song titled "He Ain't Heavy." There are so many fundraising events and activities to help animals, cancer research, diabetes research and many others. These are all worthy causes. What I have noticed is that our youth and children who are in need of help and guidance are not getting the same attention.

I have volunteered for the homeless and run-away children and have spoken with them about what they have experienced in life and how they got to where they are. It is not pretty. One kid responded to my question about how he came to the special home that was taking care of him. He responded, "My mother didn't want me." I had a hard time maintaining my composure as he was sharing his story with me. Why am I sharing this? I want to encourage you to donate time and / or money to help our youth, especially our troubled youth that need help getting back on track.

Here are some resources to help our youth:

The Covenant House
www.coveanthouse.org

Sheridan House
www.sheridanhouse.org

Books and Other Products by
Lt. Co onel. Bob Weinstein, USAR-Ret.
www.BeachBootCamp.net

Boot Camp Fitness for All Shapes and Sizes
Paperback, $19.95, 265 pages, ISBN 978-0-9841783-1-5
EBook, $9.95, ISBN 978-0-984-17837-7 (all formats)

Food & Fitness Journal
Paperback, $14.95, 212 pages, ISBN 978-1-935759-03-4
EBook, $4.95, ISBN 978-1-935759-05-8 (all formats)

Weight Loss - Twenty Pounds in Ten Weeks
Paperback, $18.95, 220 pages, ISBN 978-0-9841783-0-8
EBook, $9.99, ISBN 978-0-984-17834-6 (all formats)

Quotes to Live By
Paperback, $11.95, ISBN 978-0-9841783-2-2
EBook, $5.95, ISBN 978-0-984-17833-9 (all formats)

Discover Your Inner Strength (co-author)
Paperback, $19.95
Ebook, $9.95, ISBN 978-0-984-17836-0 (pdf)

Six Keys to Permanent Weight Loss
Audio book as MP3 download (Amazon), 60 minutes
$6.93

Eight Secrets to Longevity, Health and Fitness
Audio book as MP3 download (Amazon), 50 minutes
$8.91

Health Colonel Boot Camp T-Shirts, Mugs, etc.
Go to www.cafepress.com/healthcolonel to order online

Other books by Health Colonel Publishing

The Tale of the Little Duckling by Grit Weinstein
Paperback, $14.95, picture book story for 4 to 8 year olds
ISBN 978-0-9841783-8-4
EBook, $5.99, ISBN 978-0-984-17839-1 (all formats)

Lollopy Goes Olympic by Grit Weinstein
Paperback, $14.95, picture book for 4 to 8 year old
ISBN 978-1-935759-06-5
EBook, $5.95, ISBN 978-1-935759-07-2

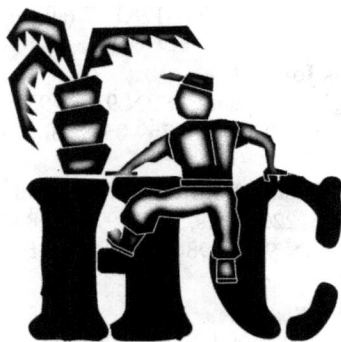

THEHEALTHCOLONEL.COM

CHANGING THE WAY PEOPLE
THINK ABOUT HEALTH.

QUICK ORDER FORM
Or order anywhere books are sold online or in store
www.BeachBootCamp.net

Fax orders: 866-481-2804. Send this form.

Telephone orders: Call 954-636-5351

Email orders: thehealthcolonel@beachbootcamp.net

Postal orders: The Health Colonel, Lt. Col. Bob Weinstein, USAR-Ret.,
757 SE 17th Street, #267, Fort Lauderdale, FL 33316,
Telephone 954-636-5351

Please send the following books, audio CDs, DVDs:

Please send more FREE information on:

Other books   Speaking/seminars

Fitness Boot Camp   Mailing Lists

Name:

Address:

City: State: Zip:

Telephone:

Email address:
Sales tax: Please add Florida sales tax for products shipped to Florida
addresses.
Shipping:
U.S.: $4.50 for first book, CD or DVD and $2.50 for each additional product.
International: $9.50 for first product; $5.50 for each additional product
(estimate).

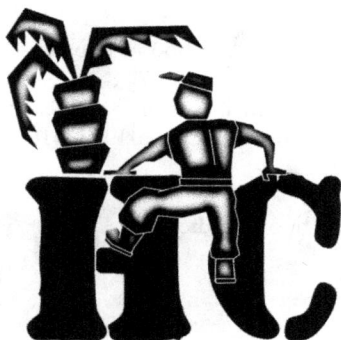

THEHEALTHCOLONEL.COM

CHANGING THE WAY PEOPLE
THINK ABOUT HEALTH.

QUICK ORDER FORM
Or order anywhere books are sold online or in store
www.BeachBootCamp.net

Fax orders: 866-481-2804. Send this form.

Telephone orders: Call 954-636-5351

Email orders: thehealthcolonel@beachbootcamp.net

Postal orders: The Health Colonel, Lt. Col. Bob Weinstein, USAR-Ret., 757 SE 17th Street, #267, Fort Lauderdale, FL 33316, Telephone 954-636-5351

Please send the following books, audio CDs, DVDs:

Please send more FREE information on:

      Other books   Speaking/seminars

      Fitness Boot Camp   Mailing Lists

Name:

Address:

City: State: Zip:

Telephone:

Email address:
Sales tax: Please add Florida sales tax for products shipped to Florida addresses.
Shipping:
U.S.: $4.50 for first book, CD or DVD and $2.50 for each additional product.
International: $9.50 for first product; $5.50 for each additional product (estimate).